Confronting Drunk Driving

Confronting Drunk Driving

Social Policy for Saving Lives

H. Laurence Ross

Foreword by Joseph R. Gusfield

Yale University Press   New Haven and London

This work was supported by the Insurance Institute for Highway Safety. The opinions, findings, and conclusions expressed in this book are those of the author and do not necessarily reflect the views of the Insurance Institute for Highway Safety.

Designed by Sonia L. Scanlon
Set in Times Roman type by Rainsford Type, Danbury, Connecticut.
Printed in the United States of America by
Vail-Ballou Press, Binghamton, New York.

Library of Congress
Cataloging-in-Publication Data

Ross, H. Laurence (Hugh Laurence)
Confronting drunk driving : social policy for saving lives / H. Laurence Ross ; foreword by Joseph R. Gusfield.
p. cm.
Includes bibliographical references and index.
ISBN 0-300-05456-4 (alk. paper)
1. Drinking and traffic accidents—Government policy. 2. Drunk driving—Government policy. I. Title.
HE5620.D7R668 1992
363.12′51—dc20   91-37598
                                   CIP

The paper in this book meets the guidelines for permanence and durability of the Committee on Production Guidelines for Book Longevity of the Council on Library Resources.

10 9 8 7 6 5 4 3 2 1

To Mark and Jeff

Contents

Foreword

Laws against drinking and driving began to appear in American society almost as soon as the automobile itself began to appear on American roads and streets. An intuitive belief existed then as now that it was risky to combine alcohol and the operation of so dangerous a vehicle. Since the end of the 1930s a complex literature of research and more than five decades of law-enforcement have created a rich body of experience, knowledge, and expertise in the understanding of traffic risks and of "drunk driving" as one of those risks. For most of the public, however, the perception of "drunk driving" is set in the context of a morality play in which the bad guys are irresponsible drunks who kill and injure the good guys, sober motorists, innocent children, and careful pedestrians. The intuitive sense of the auto as a dangerous instrument and of alcohol use as potentially hazardous has been encased in the framework in which issues of traffic safety are experienced and thought about. It is this frame that H. Laurence Ross calls the dominant paradigm.

The disposition to dramatize and simplify human issues, to personalize and crystallize them into interesting stories dominates the reporting of drinking-driving, as it does that of many other American social problems. The televised dramatization of Candy Lightner's tragic loss of her daughter in an accident involving a drunk driver was a galvanizing event in the current movement led by MADD and other organizations. These groups aim to diminish traffic fatalities largely through laws that increase the severity of punishment for drinking and driving. This approach has much in common with the prevalent public wisdom about drinking and driving, a wisdom that Ross expertly challenges in this significant volume. He shows how atypical is much of the media's dramatic rendition of traffic problems. He exposes the reader to the many other frameworks for understanding drinking-driving and to an array of alternative policies for decreasing the hazards of automobile use.

It is the immense value of this book that it challenges the dominant paradigm, in which policy proposals for auto safety are focused almost exclusively on the driver and on achieving safety through the threat of legal punishment. Ross shows his readers the limited value of such measures in preventing the dangerous outcomes of automobile use and abuse.

There is a dual dimension to public policies, which this study underscores. On one level the public discussion of drinking-driving, as of many other public problems, is a performance. Its ritualistic character is a way of asserting the moral values and ethical choices that are presented as the dominant norms of American life. It is a statement about who the good guys and who the bad guys are. In another dimension, public policies are instruments for reaching goals. The aim of traffic policy is avoidance of risk and danger, wherever found. It is important that we not confuse the ritualistic nature of public acts with their expediental ones; that we not confuse retribution and revenge with practical attainments. Saving lives and saving souls may not be the same game.

Ross is exceptionally able to challenge the conventional wisdom of the public drinking-driving discussion. He brings to the study of drinking-driving the general perspective and interest of a sociologist who has studied the process of social control through law. This provides him with a wider vision of contexts in which to perceive issues of traffic safety and automobile abuse. Coupled with this background are his many years of research and writing on general issues of deterrence through law enforcement and on drinking-driving as a special case of a dominant paradigm that stresses punishment as a deterrent. Beginning in 1960 with a major paper on traffic law violations as a "folk crime," H. Laurence Ross has produced a large body of research and writing on the topic of drinking-driving. He has also written a major study of insurance settlements, *Settled Out of Court*. His study of the outcomes of the British Road Safety Act of 1967, published in 1973, is a classic in this field. He concluded that, without continuous enforcement and reporting of that enforcement, such laws lose their initial effectiveness over time. His book *Deterring the Drinking Driver* (1982) remains a major statement of research on the subject and the leading work in the field. Throughout the present volume, Ross demonstrates his deep knowledge of the state of the art of research on drinking and driving.

What is vital to this book is the perspective of the sociologist and the expert brought to bear on the assumptions and policies of conventional wisdom. As in much of American public life, that wisdom is fundamentally psychological. By that I mean that it is oriented to understanding events as outcomes of individual choice and action. In thinking about drinking-driving, it leads to emphasis on the psychology and attributes of the motorist. A sociological perspective is attuned to contexts, to the total institutional and cultural scene that limits or expands the possibilities of crashes and the opportunities to drink and drive or not to do so. Where the psychologist sees the individual—the agent—the sociologist sees the context—the scene.

As Ross indicates in what he calls the challenging paradigm, a sociological perspective raises questions and develops policy that widen the understanding of traffic safety and increase the spectrum of measures to lower the level of loss brought about by the use of the automobile. Given the institutionally supported sale and consumption of alcohol and the widespread dependence on the auto, drinking-driving seems inevitable. Policies need to broach ways of diminishing dangerous consumption, of redesigning safer autos, of providing alternative forms of transportation, of creating more "user-friendly" roads, and other suggestions that proceed from focusing on elements other than the character of the driver.

Underlying the dual paradigms of drinking-driving and the psychological-sociological oppositions are aspects of American culture. Americans place a high value on individualism. They see the world as malleable to individual will and responsive to choice and moral character. It is to the individual that Americans so frequently look in placing responsibility for social problems. It is the base assumption that supports the great faith we have that punishing the bad guys, the drivers, will deter drinking-driving in a society whose social institutions deter public transportation and support drinking practices with limited constraints.

Sociological perspectives gain less support from those aspects of

American culture that might accept communal and institutional responsibility. To "see" events as outgrowths of more complex social institutions requires a particular way of understanding, a paradigm less individualistic than the psychological. It is less reassuring than the tacit belief that accidents are the outcome of immoral people rather than of complex, morally ambiguous, even morally acceptable actions and persons. There is a deeply held belief among Americans that the world is inherently a safe place and only the existence of evil people accounts for tragedies.

The prevailing wisdom of the public world is reinforced by mass media portrayals and official, political assertions about law enforcement and punishment. Challenging this "common sense" constitutes the impressive and unique value of Ross's attempt to place the discussion of drinking-driving in another frame of thinking. There are significant barriers that intensify the dominant paradigm and make alternative ones less appealing. The psychological assumptions and the punishment and deterrence doctrines are not only intuitive in American culture. They are also less costly. By placing all responsibility on individuals we avoid the political and economic conflicts attendant on examining our institutions, our culture, and our technological assumptions. While punishment and law enforcement are expensive, they avoid the trauma of changing our social system.

The value of this book is that it may make the reader reexamine assumptions and easy solutions to public problems. It is a virtue of the sociological perspective that it can widen the horizons of our thought and bring freshness and breadth to the narrowed and stale arenas of American social problems. H. Laurence Ross does this admirably and, one hopes, will lift the issue of drinking-driving onto a more rational and yet more imaginative level.

Joseph Gusfield

Preface

My initial research in the area of drunk driving was a product of an interest in what could be learned about the ways in which law controls behavior. Drunk driving seemed to offer important research opportunities for two reasons. First, it was the focus of numerous interventions intended to deter through the mechanism of legal threat. Second, the amount of drunk driving was relatively well measured among criminal behaviors. Although direct measurement is difficult and expensive, valid and reliable indexes such as nighttime fatalities are frequently available. New techniques of intervention analysis facilitate raising and answering questions concerning the deterrent effect of various laws. It is thus possible to explore both the potential and limits of legal control in general through studying attempts to control drunk driving.

In my first book on the topic, *Deterring the Drinking Driver*, I reviewed what had been learned by the research community in various countries over several decades with the intention of completing my contribution to the question and moving on to other things. However, the rise of the citizens' movement, leading to demands for information on what works in controlling drunk driving, pulled me into the policy dialogue.

One influence on my subsequent thinking, expressed in this second book on drunk driving, was experience with the policy-making process. I felt the frustration of testifying that effective deterrence required increases in the swiftness and certainty of punishment rather than in its severity, while people who purportedly listened to me pushed on with programs centered on mandatory jail and other severe punishments—programs that appeared to yield less than optimal results. Moreover, as someone who views the world as a fundamentally tragic place, I was distressed to see purported humanitarians adding to the amount of pain and suffering experienced by humanity with the claimed but questionable justification of deterrent accomplishments.

I have also been influenced by living in the Scandinavian countries. My research there began with an interest in criminal law as applied to drunk driving, but experience led me to an interest in policies regarding alcohol and transportation. The Scandinavian countries seem to have achieved some control over drunk driving, but not just through their criminal laws. More central to this accomplishment, in my opinion, is recognition of the causes of drunk driving in social institutions, leading to countermeasures based in alcohol policy—reducing drinking—and transportation policy—reducing driving.

Another important influence on my thought has been twenty years of association with the Insurance Institute for Highway Safety, where thinking has consistently stressed the limitations of interventions intended to change human behavior, compared with those measures that engineer an environment in which behavior as given is less likely to produce undesirable results. The time for writing this book was provided in a grant from the Institute, and its research staff were important collaborators and critics. However, although this work reflects their input, the opinions and recommendations offered here are mine and are not necessarily endorsed by the Institute.

I wish to express my deep appreciation to the colleagues who have now and over the years helped me to think through the issues addressed in this book. Special thanks are due to those people at the Institute who read every chapter as it was completed and responded with helpful criticism: Brian O'Neill, Allan Williams, and Adrian Lund. Steve Bloch, Jim McKnight, and Bob Voas likewise offered extensive comments on every chapter. Joe Gusfield evaluated the manuscript for Yale and wrote the splendid Foreword. Among other people offering valuable advice in specific areas were Michele Fields, Mark Freedman, Chuck Hurley, and Paul Zador at the Institute, along with Joel Best, Louise Caffin, Jim Fell, Jim Frank, Frank Haight, Mark Hauswald, Jim Jacobs, Hans Klette, Susan Lockhart, John McCarthy, Joan Quinlan, Pat Taylor, and Alex Wagenaar. The services of the Institute's library staff—especially Kris Pruzin and Sharon Hoffman—were essential to this work and were cheerfully and efficiently provided.

Finally, I wish to acknowledge the encouragement of my work by the citizens' movement against drunk driving. Although I have at times felt frustrated by the unwillingness of movement organizations to follow certain promising paths, I recognize we have somewhat different agendas, moderately different political stances, and sometimes vastly different views of the world, including assumptions about the nature of human behavior. Where we unite is in our concern with saving lives now lost due to drunk driving. I hope that the members of Remove Intoxicated Drivers and Mothers Against Drunk Driving and other groups will find this book relevant and challenging. Without the movement's incessant and impassioned activity, drunk driving would not be a matter of national concern, nor would many people choose to read this book.

Confronting Drunk Driving

Introduction

This book is about saving lives. More accurately, it is about prolonging lives, specifically those at risk in alcohol-related highway crashes. It offers an array of policy options for reducing the numbers of deaths and injuries caused by driving while impaired by alcohol or, to use the prevailing label, drunk driving.

The American drunk driving problem has been recognized, defined, and addressed with some success by policies based on the view that what is at issue is criminal behavior pure and simple, controllable by means of the criminal justice system. This view, the "dominant paradigm" by which drunk driving is understood, has up to now controlled the policy agenda for dealing with drunk driving in America. It has led to countermeasures which, though successful to some degree, seem restricted in their impact. Moreover, the commitments needed in order to enact the policies in effect today have to some extent trapped their advocates and made it difficult for them to accept the possibility that although some policies may be working well, others are inefficient and even ineffective. Taking a broad sociological and evaluative view of the drunk driving problem will point to avenues for maximizing the impact of current strategies. It will also permit consideration of new countermeasures capable of saving additional lives.

A decade has passed since I addressed the issue of what to do about drunk driving in my book *Deterring the Drinking Driver: Legal Policy and Social Control*. This decade has been one of great activity in the development and application of innovative policies for confronting drunk driv-

1

ing. Many of the innovations have been accompanied by evaluations, some extensive and informative. Much more is known about what can and cannot be accomplished in reducing drunk driving, especially with deterrence-based measures. In addition, new political actors have developed a concern with the drunk driving problem. Medical and public health interests have entered the fray of drunk driving politics with a "challenging paradigm" for understanding the problem, which has led to new ideas for countermeasures. I have tried to utilize this paradigm in proposing policy options for the further saving of lives.

A lifesaving approach to the drunk driving problem

There is broad consensus that a drunk driving problem exists in America. Its nature and size are matters of conventional, though debatable, understanding. Drivers who are drunk, in the sense of being visibly and extremely intoxicated, are blamed for the loss of as many as twenty-five thousand lives in highway crashes each year and hundreds of thousands of severe injuries. The drunk drivers are understood to have long histories of prior arrests for similar behavior. In contrast, most of those killed and injured are believed to be innocent victims whose behavior did not contribute to their deaths. The drunk driving problem, it is believed, could be largely avoided if the criminal justice system did its job in punishing offenders.

Yet crash data suggest that the conventional understanding of the drunk driving problem is partial and misleading and that this distortion affects the policies that are intended to ameliorate the problem. For instance, the number of deaths caused by drunk driving is considerably smaller than the number of alcohol-related traffic fatalities, and even in crashes clearly involving alcohol impairment as a causal factor the stereotypical drunk driver is seldom found. Contrary to the impression that the drunk driver has a long criminal record before he kills, the vast majority of those killing in alcohol-related crashes have no known prior convictions for drunk driving. Finally, despite the belief that drunk drivers usually kill innocent people, most of the drunk drivers' victims are the drivers themselves, their often drunken passengers, and drunken pedestrians and cyclists. These facts do not reduce the tragedy of drunk driving, but they caution against uncritical acceptance of the picture painted in conventional discourse as well as undue reliance on countermeasures that are narrowly directed to the conventional image.

The term *drunk driving* is not a felicitous one to describe the problem

2

as referenced by the above facts. A more grammatical and less misleading term would be *alcohol-impaired driving*. This acknowledges the fact that an increased risk of a serious crash occurs with all but the most minimal concentrations of alcohol in the blood of drivers. The risk, though accelerating with increasing blood alcohol, shows no point of inflection at which to divide "safe" drinking and driving from "drunk" drinking and driving. If, given these facts, I still refer to the problem as drunk driving, it is because social problems, including their designations, are created by consensus. One must use the term in order to participate in the relevant debate.

Policy for reducing drunk driving has traditionally centered on deterrence through criminal law. Deterrence employs a threat of punishment to change the balance of outcomes for specific behavior. It thus depends for its success on people's perception and evaluation of the rewards and sanctions obtainable from different courses of behavior. This approach has comprised the center of current policies partly because punishment seems to be exceptionally appropriate for people who are seen as choosing to impose the consequences of their negligent and risky behavior on other people.

Many legal threats have turned out over time to lack credibility, and thus a deterrent impact, because of a low objective risk of apprehension and punishment for law violators. However, with sufficient resources some deterrent threats can be rendered credible, to the point of reducing law violations and saving lives. Moreover, deterrent policies may eventually affect related social norms, countering the incentives people have to drink and drive with external sanctions of shame and internal ones of guilt, in addition to legal sanctions.

Yet deterrence has inherent limits as a tool for reducing drunk driving. It does not address the social causes of impaired driving. Although some individuals may decide on specific occasions to refrain from drinking and driving because of the deterrent threat, the underlying causes continue to produce incentives to drink and drive that are hard to resist, even when they are reinforced by the threat of punishment.

Relatively little recent political discussion has paid attention to these causal factors. Attention has focused on which individuals are likely to accumulate arrests and crashes and how to affect that decision. It has not inquired about what determines the numbers and rates of alcohol-related crash fatalities, why these seem in some sense to be exceptionally high in America, and how the rates might be lowered.

These issues can be addressed by a sociological analysis, which looks for social factors as influences on or determinants of behavior.

The social causes of drunk driving in America lie in a conjunction of institutions. American society combines a near-total commitment to private automobile transportation with a positive evaluation of drinking in recreational situations. Conventional and conforming behavior in these areas implies the likelihood of people driving while impaired by alcohol. Furthermore, in certain social categories, such as younger males, the norms regarding both drinking and driving appear to be extraordinarily favorable for the creation of impaired driving. Drunk driving can thus be seen as a routine, expected aspect of American life, supported by prevailing norms and institutions. This characterization applies in general and even more in particular subgroups.

To the extent this analysis is convincing, drunk driving should be influenced by policies that reduce the overall use of cars and of alcohol as well as by those specifically addressed to the intersection of these uses. Prohibitions such as minimum ages for drinking and for driving and intrusions in the market for alcohol and automobiles, exemplified by taxes and regulations, illustrate the potential for such policies. Research demonstrates the ability of many such measures to reduce drunk driving, and possibly this immediate success can encourage a view of drinking and driving that renders it less socially acceptable over time. This effect has been posited for the criminal law, and it seems plausible for regulatory laws as well.

Another policy approach for dealing with the deaths and injuries caused by drunk driving is through attenuating the links between impairment and error and crashes, and between crashes and injuries and deaths. Thus, deaths due to drunk driving can be reduced without necessarily decreasing the amount of impairment. Examples of this approach are found in highway and vehicle engineering and in improved emergency medical services.

The policy agenda offered in this book is not simple. Drunk driving, like many other social problems, resists simple solutions. The proposals form a package that approaches the problem in a variety of ways, each of which is capable of contributing to its reduction. The package is offered with the goal of reducing the problem, not eliminating it. Because drunk driving is built into basic social institutions and to some degree even into the physical structure of American communities, its elimination seems an unrealistic goal. What is more, effective countermeasures entail costs, including those of renouncing some benefits that many people assume are part of the American life-style. Policies that promise important progress in reducing drunk driving at little or no cost must be regarded as unrealistic, if not fraudulent.

The causes of drunk driving

The basic insight of this book is that drunk driving in America, understood as encompassing all driving during which the risk of a serious crash is importantly elevated by alcohol, is a predictable product of our social institutions, especially transportation and recreation. On the one hand, we live in a society that assumes the widespread use of private automotive transportation for all daily functions, including work, shopping, worship, medical care, and recreation. On the other hand, we accept as appropriate the use of alcohol in a variety of common activities, especially those defined as integral to leisure and recreation. If we are less likely today than in the past to accept the three-martini business lunch, we still believe that "beer belongs" when people relax after the close of business. In many circles, the quantities and frequencies of expected alcohol consumption are sufficient to produce considerable impairment of driving-related faculties. The conjunction of these social institutions goes far to explain the existence and entrenchment of the drunk driving problem in America.

The dependence of Americans on the private automobile is extreme, and in some situations virtually total. Except in the largest cities, alternatives to automobile transportation are inconvenient, expensive, unpleasant, dangerous, or nonexistent. More than four out of five trips of all types in the United States are made in privately owned motor vehicles. In recent years, these vehicles have traveled nearly 2 trillion (2,000 billion) miles. The extent of our automobile dependence is suggested by the fact that possession of a driver's license is nearly universal. Indeed, it can be said that the license serves as a kind of national identity card. Moreover, the availability of cars has transformed even the physical structure of American society so that driving has become to all intents and purposes a necessity.

The use of alcohol is almost equally ingrained in American society. Alcohol is overwhelmingly accepted as a facilitator of sociable interaction, and the great majority of adults drink. Most drinking can be regarded as moderate, or social, drinking, which is conventionally considered harmless and compatible with safe driving. However, social drinking is often sufficient to produce a doubling or more of the risk of a serious crash if combined with driving. In addition, many social circles accept and encourage heavy drinking, which multiplies the risk of serious crashes by factors in the hundreds. Just as we can assume that for a large fraction of the public all activities outside the home involve driving, so we can assume that for most people leisure activities are likely to involve drinking, sometimes heavy drinking. Putting these assumptions together, we note that for a significant fraction of Americans drinking and driving represents a "natural" conjunction of activities. The drunk driving problem, as broadly defined in this writing, is thus seen to be intimately integrated with the American life-style.

The consequences of drunk driving

Chapter 2 of this book reviews the implications of the conjunction of institutions discussed here for the lives and deaths of Americans. It will be seen that the presence of measurable amounts of alcohol in the bodies of drivers is statistically and causally associated with increased probabilities of highway crashes, especially of the more serious ones involving injuries and fatalities. This is perhaps obvious after years of media attention. What is not so obvious is that the increased risk of a crash, especially of a serious one, begins with relatively low amounts of alcohol in the body, including those that can result from moderate drinking. Other things being equal, increased consumption results in increased crash risk, and the relationship accelerates with heavier drinking. Recent research suggests that at a blood-alcohol concentration (BAC) of 0.05 percent, which could be reached by an average person drinking two or three standard drinks (e.g., a 12-ounce glass of beer, a 4-ounce glass of wine, or 1 ½ ounces of whiskey) within an hour on an empty stomach, the fatal crash risk is doubled. At around 0.08 percent, attainable by some people with three or four drinks, the risk is multiplied by ten; at 0.10 percent, the legal limit in most states, the risk may be multiplied by more than twenty; and at BACs over 0.15 percent, typically attained by persons arrested for drunk driving, the risk is multiplied by hundreds. These ratios, calculated from data on actual crashes, are supported and explained by laboratory investigations of the effects of alcohol on driving-related skills.

The increased risk of crashes caused by alcohol impairment creates a large pool of deaths and injuries, which is central to the perception of drunk driving as a social problem. However, the contribution of alcohol to deaths and injuries derives not from its rendering each individual trip disastrous, but rather by increasing the crash risk per mile traveled. The resultant increased risk, though still small in an absolute sense, when applied to the enormous mileage accumulated by American drivers produces consequences that can be regarded as disastrous in the aggregate. Moreover, the deaths associated with highway crashes result in an extraordinary number of potential years of life lost, owing to the relatively young age of those killed in crashes compared with those affected by other common causes of death. The drunk driving problem is made more poignant—and the demand for countermeasures more urgent—because of the youth of those involved.

Deterrence-based countermeasures

Deterrence, or the threat of legal punishment for drunk driving, has been the focus of most contemporary policy addressing drunk driving. This approach is reviewed in chapter 3. The centerpiece of the deterrent approach to behavior in general and drunk driving in particular is the proposition that behavior will be altered or abandoned to the extent that it is threatened with what is perceived as certain, swift, and severe punishment. The expectation is indifferent to the causes of the behavior in question. Deterrence is not concerned with stemming the desire or motivation to commit the threatened act. The deterrent approach seeks instead to burden the prohibited act with sufficient negative consequences to constrain the potential delinquent from committing it.

Because deterrent threats, if they are effective, can usually be expected to have immediate consequences, their accomplishments in the short run are capable of evaluation if the behavior in question can be well measured. Traffic law in general and drunk driving law in particular have been among the most active areas of deterrence research. This is because of the relatively reliable and valid indexes of effectiveness available at low cost in data on serious crashes, as well as the proliferation of natural experiments entailed in crackdowns on traffic offenders generally and drunk drivers particularly.

The deterrence proposition can be seen as a restatement of the law of demand in economics. Predictions based on that law have been repeatedly supported in market-based research by economists, and it would be surprising if it were found to be totally without confirmation in nonmarket settings, including the attempt to reduce crime in general and drunk driving in particular. Indeed, review of the proliferating literature on drunk driving supports the expectation that deterrent threats can have results and that we are currently benefiting from these. However, not all aspects of the deterrence proposition have been confirmed.

The key to effective deterrence of drunk driving (and other crimes as well) appears to lie in the perception of swift and certain punishment more than in perceived severity. Indeed, there is considerable evidence that increasing the objective severity of the threat in a situation of very low objective likelihood of punishment is often ineffective. Moreover, if the threat is evaluated by those charged with its application as disproportionate in severity to the harm involved, that is, unfair, the officials may refrain from applying it. Thus, a severe threat may have the unintended and unanticipated consequence of reducing the likelihood of any punishment at all for the behavior in question.

Chapter 3 expands my previous review of experience in attempting drunk driving deterrence. The conclusions remain the same: successful deterrent countermeasures are those that promise swift and certain punishment, rather than those that increase punishment severity. Measures such as mandatory jail terms and unusually long license revocations are generally ineffective in reducing drunk driving. In contrast, investments in law enforcement are frequently rewarded with reductions in drunk driving.

My conclusion is that properly designed deterrent measures are capable of effectively reducing drunk driving. However, their achievements require appropriate enforcement efforts and resources. Deterrent laws do not jump off the statute book pages and apply themselves; and deterrent measures leave the basic recreational and transportation practices underlying drunk driving largely untouched. Even given their documented success when properly applied, the problem they address can and should be further affected by countermeasures based on modifying its social causes.

Countermeasures based in alcohol policy

Chapter 4 surveys those countermeasures that are expected to reduce drunk driving by reducing the amount that people drink, both overall and especially in places generally reached by car. Such policies can be divided into those increasing the price of alcoholic beverages and those reducing availability. A few policies focus on affecting social incentives to drink specifically in conjunction with driving.

Although these policies have sometimes been referred to as "neo-Prohibitionistic," the label seems unjust. It is true that a principal lesson of past alcohol prohibitions in the United States and elsewhere has been that it is possible to use law successfully to reduce both alcohol consumption and related problems. However, general prohibitions are acknowledged to be costly in several senses. The costs include depriving people of what many define as pleasurable and desirable experiences. There are no serious proposals today for resuscitating general alcohol prohibitions. Moreover, the prohibitions of the past have been based on a moralistic condemnation of alcohol which has led to an unnecessary extremism in their scope and enforcement. A less moralistic alcohol policy might aim for effective and acceptable means of minimizing the negative consequences of alcohol use, which are usually a function of the frequent consumption of high quantities, while retaining the positive ones, which are likely to be associated with occasional and moderate consumption. It is not necessary to consider alcohol an evil substance in order to see dangers in its use and to posit the need for policies regulating the conditions under which it is consumed.

Alcohol-based policies include what has been among the most effective recent countermeasures to drunk driving: the minimum drinking age, which imposes prohibition on a limited group of young adults. Although considerations of equity may temper enthusiasm for a drinking age higher than the age of adulthood, research shows that this countermeasure has been dramatically effective in reducing drunk driving among the population to which it applies. Its success argues for the promise of other possible countermeasures based in alcohol policy.

A related example of countermeasures to drunk driving based in alcohol policy is excise taxation of beverages for the purpose of increasing their price and thus diminishing their consumption. The tool might cut more finely if taxes could be related to the relative dangerousness of the consumption in question, for example, in the form of a surtax on beverages sold in locations where subsequent driving is especially likely.

Reducing the availability of alcohol through the regulation of sales and service practices is another possible strategy for reducing drunk driving. The relationship between numbers of outlets and the extent of drunk driving is not a simple one, and indiscriminate elimination of sales points is unlikely to be effective. However, numerous serving practices that appear to encourage excessive drinking might be restricted. Examples are solicitation of drink orders by service personnel ("pushing" drinks), the requirement of a minimum purchase where entertainment is provided, and promotions such as half-price "happy hours" and "drink-and-drown" nights, during which unlimited consumption is permitted for a fixed price. Research supports the effectiveness of some such regulation. Another possibility is training servers to recognize impairment and tactfully to deflect alcohol consumption by some part of the clientele. Research indicates that this training is capable of changing knowledge, although behavior change may be limited in the face of ambivalent management policies.

Finally, in this category, promotion and marketing practices could be evaluated and restrained to the extent that they seem likely to increase alcohol consumption, especially in conjunction with driving. Recommendations of this type must face the fact that direct scientific evidence of a link between beverage advertising and consumption has proved elusive. Some such link can be inferred, however, both from commonsense observation and from general social science evidence concerning the influence of communications on behavior.

Countermeasures based in transportation policy

Chapter 5 surveys those drunk driving countermeasures that address the problem through changes in the means of transportation. These opportunities in general have been less salient in recent policy debates than those based on changes in drinking. The neglect is understandable, for the automobile in general lacks the ambivalent or even negative symbolism that is frequently associated with alcohol in America, and societal commitment to automotive transportation is generally unquestioned. However, the potential for saving lives through reducing the use of private automobiles is real, even though many of the specific countermeasures can be expected to be implemented only in the long run. One example of such a measure would be a taxi subsidy during drinking hours, in order to induce people to ride both to and from drinking sites. Related policies include designated driver programs sponsored by the beverage industry, the "contract for life" (and alternative transportation home) sponsored by Students Against Driving Drunk (SADD), and safe rides or "tipsy taxi" programs, which provide one-way rides home for bar patrons whom management judges to be intoxicated. These programs have seldom been competently evaluated, and they appear to be underused where offered—but many of them make sense intuitively and in theory.

As a parallel to the minimum drinking age, an increase in the minimum age for driving, especially during drinking hours, could be expected to have an effect on drunk driving by reducing exposure of a group with an unusually high alcohol-related crash rate. In the few states presently restricting nighttime driving by young people, rates of crashes among teenagers are lower than in comparable states lacking such curfews.

Saving lives in spite of drunk driving

From the public health perspective that characterizes this book, drunk driving is problematic mainly to the extent that it leads to death and injury. Were the roads to be populated with drunk drivers who caused no deaths or injuries, the situation would warrant less concern (though other health problems associated with long-term excessive use of alcohol would still have to be addressed). From the traffic safety viewpoint, drunk driving might be tolerable if its links to errors and crashes, and subsequently to injuries and deaths, could be severed. The total severance of these links is unlikely, but an attenuation of their strength could be considered an important accomplishment. Several ways of effecting these changes are detailed in chapter 6.

A first approach in this category focuses on the link between impairment and driver error. Engineering knowledge furnishes numerous examples of how the driving task may be simplified and thus rendered less likely to be botched because of impairment. In addition, technology can attenuate the link between errors and crashes. Examples can be offered in vehicle and highway design improvements.

The link between crashes and injuries may be addressed through technology that reduces the severity of crashes that do take place. For example, roadside hazards can be buffered or weakened within limits, and guardrails and breakaway utility poles can be installed. The proportion of crashes that injure or kill can also be reduced by measures that center on engineering the vehicle to reduce the forces experienced by passengers' bodies in their collisions with structures inside the car. Seat belts are demonstrably effective when used, and mandatory use laws and incentive programs appear capable of realizing important increments in their use. A notable recent development has been the installation of air bags, which are truly passive and do not require any affirmative behavior by vehicle occupants in order to be effective. Finally, deaths can be reduced and injuries lessened by providing appropriate medical care to injured parties at the earliest possible time. Emergency medical services probably deserve some credit for the improving mileage-based crash death rates of the last several years.

A general advantage of measures that affect the consequences of behavior rather than the behavior itself is that no changes in basic social values are required. Although such measures have been perhaps least salient in the current social response to drunk driving, in some ways they may be seen as the most acceptable of all approaches in that they save lives without challenging institutions.

A policy agenda

This book is written with the understanding that social problems are political constructs. They are defined and typified by a political process in which science is only peripherally involved, and they are attacked with countermeasures that are also politically vetted. It is the intent of this book to widen the definition of the drunk driving problem in America to include all driving that occurs when skills and abilities are significantly impaired by alcohol. Furthermore, I hope to encourage the perception that drunk driving, tragic and harmful as it is, is not an isolated problem, but that it represents an intersection between two much larger and even more menacing sources of death and injury—traffic crashes and alcohol problems.

Drunk driving is not a puzzling or arbitrary phenomenon. Its causes can be seen as situated in the conjunction of institutions noted here. Some promising countermeasures are thus likely to involve changing the institutions. However, such change cannot be accomplished without costs, very likely including those of relinquishing benefits obtained from accepted institutional arrangements. Institutional change is seldom easy, but when its benefits are perceived to overwhelm the costs it would seem feasible and worthwhile.

Other effective policies may obviate the need for major change in our daily habits. One of these is deterrence. On the one hand, the costs of deterrence should not be underestimated: appearances sometimes to the contrary, successful deterrence is not free. On the other hand, its potential for saving lives ought not to be denigrated. Also in this category is the cluster of measures that aim at vitiating the links between impairment and death. Their costs are usually self-evident, but their benefits may well outweigh the costs.

In chapter 7 I offer a policy agenda for dealing with drunk driving. It consists in part of techniques known to be effective. Some of these, such as mandating a high minimum drinking age, are already in effect and yield lifesaving benefits at the present time; they merely require attention and enforcement. Others, such as increasing the price of alcoholic beverages, rest on a strong knowledge base. However, their optimal form is not known and cannot be known without experience. A further category, including such measures as subsidizing taxi service, consists of unproved but plausible opportunities that merit exploration through pilot programs and scientific evaluations.

This listing includes items from all approaches reviewed in this book— deterrence of drunk driving, reducing drinking, reducing driving, and attenuating the links between impairment and deaths. All are capable of making a contribution to saving lives, and none should be over- looked.

My view is strongly affected by the belief that the bottom line for social policy is extending and improving lives, without regard to the nature of the particular hazard that imperils them. Drunk driving is important not of itself but because it is a major factor in shortening human lives and filling them with pain. Reducing drunk driving is a pressing social imperative because of this. However, reducing its con- sequences may be at least as important from the bottom-line perspec- tive. Resources expended on such policies as providing emergency medical services systems can be justified as drunk driving counter- measures even if they leave the extent of impairment untouched. More- over, drunk driving has to take its place in the priority line along with other sources of human suffering, and its claim for resources has to be balanced against claims related to other social problems, including the related ones of traffic safety and alcohol in general. In my view, the claims of drunk driving possess a special urgency because of the youth of so many of those who are affected; but other conditions such as drug addiction and AIDS also fall disproportionately on the young and demand priority as problems. The balance of investments in var- ious policies must reflect both the magnitude of the problems as causes of death and suffering and the efficiency and effectiveness of expend- itures made to control them. Looking only within the field of traffic safety for examples, we find that funds are wasted on imprisonment when license suspension is more capable of reducing drunk driving. We can also waste funds on quite effective countermeasures if the problem is extremely rare. This is exemplified by demands for occupant-protection devices in school buses, vehicles in which the current occupant fatality rate is virtually zero. Likewise, the proposed requirement of protective seats for infants flying in commercial aircraft is well intentioned, but the benefits are likely to be immensely costly.

Drunk driving is a major cause of deaths and injuries, and as such it merits priority in discussion and action. Although it cannot be eliminated so long as society continues to value both alcohol consumption and automotive transportation, it can be reduced by affordable countermeasures that have either been proved effective or can reasonably be deemed promising. The progress of the past decade in reducing alcohol-related deaths on the highway is welcomed, but it is not sufficient to permit complacency with regard to the tens of thousands who continue to die, and the millions who suffer, as a consequence of drunk driving in America. The understandings and countermeasures offered here are intended to be broader and more fundamental than those dominating the thinking of the past decade. Without denigrating what has been accomplished, this program is offered as a means of thinking about steps that promise effectively and efficiently to save additional lives.

Roads not taken

This book is about the social problem of drunk driving. Indirectly, it concerns both overall traffic safety and alcohol problems in general. Beyond these, I intend the reasoning to serve as a model for thinking about social problems most generally. However, the book does not attempt to deal with those larger problems in a systematic way. For example, the reader will not find a systematic discussion of theories or treatment of alcoholism, and interventions designed to deal with heavy drinking are evaluated for their impact on traffic safety, not for their usefulness in curing a disease or reformulating a problematic lifestyle. The book contains no discussion of drugs other than alcohol, even though there is a suspicion that drugs of all types, including over-the-counter and prescription medicines as well as illegal drugs, may be causal factors in some fatal crashes. Little attention is paid to alcohol-impaired pedestrians, though they represent a significant fraction of alcohol-related crash fatalities. Given the seamless web of the human condition, inclusion of these topics as related to the issues treated in the book would have been defensible. My decisions on inclusions and exclusions are largely based on the desire to address a particular social problem—drunk driving—that appears as an object of current political discourse. My regrets go to those who would have preferred a broader reach.

Causes and Consequences of Drunk Driving

When we speak of a social problem we think in terms of an objective condition that is self-evidently harmful. On reflection, however, it is clear that the objectivity of conditions is an assumption rather than an absolute truth and that harmfulness of conditions involves a subjective judgment about them. The statement that something is a social problem is most conveniently regarded as a claim put forth by some interested party. The claim refers to the existence, nature, and extent of a condition. Social problems claims usually include the idea that the condition is harmful, that it is changeable, and that government or "society" has an obligation to change it (Spector and Kitsuse, 1987; Best, 1989).

Social problems, then, may be conceived as products of a political process in which claims are raised and debated and in which greater or less consensus is achieved concerning the existence, prevalence, harmfulness, ameliorability, urgency, and other characteristics of a purported hazard. The distribution of income in society, for example, becomes the poverty problem; deviant and perplexing behavior becomes the problem of mental illness; and driving while impaired by alcohol becomes the drunk driving problem.

Social problems can come and go with little evidence of change in the real world. Heroin, for example, was a major social problem in the 1950s, but it became a minor problem in the 1960s and 1970s even though there is no evidence that consumption of the drug declined. Public attention was diverted from heroin in part because of competition from other problems like war and poverty. Heroin reemerged as a major

2

social problem because of its association with AIDS in the 1980s. Social problems can even be created through claims about conditions that are scientifically undemonstrable: consider flying saucers and witchcraft (Spector and Kitsuse, 1987).

Social problems are understood with the benefit of statistics, which depict the magnitude of the problem, and typifications, which depict the nature of the problem. Neither statistics nor typifications convey information neutrally; rather, they are part of the political process whereby selected conditions become social problems.

This understanding implies that social policies for reducing or controlling problems respond not to conditions in the real world, but to images. Analysts and critics of these policies also rely on images of conditions. These images often emerge from an agenda that differs from that of the policymakers, one in which claims of science and objectivity are put forward, but which more modest proponents will admit shares the inherently political nature of social constructs.

This book offers a critique of current drunk driving policy and develops an alternative agenda for saving lives currently lost because of impaired driving. Candor requires that I present my assumptions and agenda. The present chapter thus shares with readers my personal understanding of the nature of drinking and driving and of effective social policy.

I see the condition we call drunk driving as lying at the intersection of two broader problems—the alcohol problem and the traffic safety problem. Inclusion of drunk driving in the alcohol problem links it to numerous other types of alcohol-related violence, including murders, homicides, suicides, drownings, and the like, as well as to physical deterioration in cirrhosis, cancer, and other diseases. Inclusion of drunk driving in the traffic safety problem links it to crashes due to drugs other than alcohol (including both legal and illegal ones), fatigue, senility, inexperience, and other factors. From the viewpoint of those concerned with these larger problems, there may be little reason to single out drunk driving for special attention. For example, from the traffic safety viewpoint, why is it more important to prevent crashes caused by alcohol impairment than to prevent those—indeed, the majority—in which other factors are more prominent? Why, from the alcohol problem viewpoint, are crashes of more concern than deadly assaults? Although there are answers to these questions, they are pri-

17

marily political, not scientific. Each of the larger problems has its own social and political constituency, people who are concerned about drunk driving as an aspect of alcohol or traffic safety. However, drunk driving has an independent constituency. It has thus become established as a discrete social problem, meriting discussion and analysis on its own as well as in its larger contexts.

Since definitions are keys to understanding, this chapter offers a definition of the drunk driving problem, one that originates in but expands upon the conventional one. It then explores the evidence concerning the extent of the problem. It offers a sociologically based analysis of the causes of drunk driving and critically appraises the evidence concerning its consequences. It concludes with a summary of current trends and points to the contribution that may be expected from policies to be recommended in subsequent chapters.

A definition of drunk driving

Drunk driving is the name of a social problem; it identifies a purportedly problematic condition and demands countermeasures. While drunk driving is the problem, the condition indicated in the problem and addressed by the countermeasures is driving while impaired by alcohol to the point that the risk of a serious crash is significantly elevated. The condition does not imply clinical manifestations of drunkenness or intoxication. The issue is the dangerousness of behavior, not its obviousness or deviance.

This view of drunk driving encompasses a broader range of behavior than is usually envisaged in policy discussions. Drunk drivers are not exclusively, or even commonly, grossly intoxicated individuals whose impairment is evident in the way they smell, speak, and drive. Drunk driving as defined here includes conditions in which alteration of behavior is clinically undetectable. Indeed, these conditions are more common than not among people with significantly impairing concentrations of alcohol in their blood. *Drunk driving* may therefore be considered a misleading label, as it implies visibly deviant behavior, but this is the label that has been used to construct the contemporary American problem. An implicit acceptance of "drunk driving" without "drunkenness" in current policy is shown in the near-universal acceptance of laws that prohibit driving with more than a stipulated blood-alcohol concentration. These laws do not permit the excuse that the driver was not intoxicated, and many experienced drinkers would not, at such a concentration, present visible evidence of their impairment.

To define drunk driving as driving while significantly impaired introduces an evaluative term, *significant*. My use of this term refers not to statistical significance (the conclusion that an observed difference is due to factors other than mere chance), but to practical importance. Because the impairing effect of alcohol on driving and other behavior is variable, and because the extent to which any phenomenon is important is inherently arguable, it is difficult to offer a highly precise quantification of significance in this context. However, a rough approximation can be offered to facilitate discussion. I suggest using the blood-alcohol concentration (percentage of alcohol in the blood, or BAC) of 0.04 percent as an indication of significant impairment of driving ability by alcohol. This is the figure recommended by the Transportation Research Board (1987) and adopted by the U.S. Department of Transportation as the limit of toleration for blood alcohol applicable to commercial drivers. With BACs in this general vicinity, the risk of a fatal crash is roughly twice that of driving with no alcohol in the blood.

The figure I suggest for defining drunk driving is, of course, lower than the BAC legally tolerated in most American states (0.10 percent) or than the 0.08 percent limit now prevailing in Britain, Canada, and a few leading American jurisdictions, including California. It is even lower than the emerging European standard of 0.05 percent BAC. However, the question of what ought to be tolerated before the law steps in is rather different and more limited than the question of what degree of danger should be considered problematic and worthy of countermeasures. Law, especially criminal law, is usually a measure of last resort, not a guide to what is responsible or even sensible behavior.

It is further desirable to translate BAC, the index of impairment, into a description of drinking that can be understood in lay terms. Doing this is not easy either because BAC is a function not only of the quantity consumed but also of the consumption time, body type (gender and weight) of the drinker, quantity of food in the stomach, composition of the beverage in which alcohol is included, and other matters (Evans, 1991: 163–69). As an illustration, however, according to the Colorado Drink/Drive Calculator, people in ordinary drinking situations would on average attain a BAC of 0.04 percent after consuming, in one hour, two or three standard drinks. Among those accustomed to drinking, it is unlikely that the consequent impairment would be obvious, either to lay companions or professionals, including physicians and police. Indeed, one study of alcoholics (Perper, Twerski, and Weinand, 1986) found that a quarter of subjects with BACs of 0.20 percent or more—twice the legal limit for drivers in most states—showed no signs of clinical intoxication, such as slurred speech or unsteady gait!

An important multiple of serious crash risk for drivers at BACs around 0.04 percent is suggested by field (epidemiological) studies (Zador, 1989) and confirmed by laboratory or clinical studies of abilities related to safe driving (Moskowitz and Robinson, 1988). This is the approximate border I would draw for the drunk driving problem. However, the issue of alcohol impairment and driving extends further: "[I]nvestigators have not found an absolute threshold below which there is no [driving] impairment of any kind. Certain skills important for driving are impaired at 0.01 to 0.02 percent BAC or, in other words, at the lowest levels that can be measured reliably" (Moskowitz and Burns, 1990: 14).

The degree of danger occasioned by the driving of marginally impaired drinkers is not great in absolute terms. If alcohol-free driving is associated with about one death in 50 million vehicle miles (a plausible estimate given that the total mileage-based death rate is 2.2 per hundred million miles), the fatality rate for drivers with a doubled risk would be one in 25 million miles. Still, we can define this degree of hazard as problematic because, owing to our enormous mileage, a doubled death rate is capable of producing thousands of "unnecessary" corpses annually.

If driving with a BAC of 0.04 percent is considered problematic, driving with more elevated concentrations of alcohol is much more so. Indeed, the relationship between BAC and risk of fatal crashes increases steeply and geometrically. For example, according to Zador's (1989) calculations, a male driver aged twenty-five or over with a BAC between 0.05 and 0.09 percent has a fatality risk in single-vehicle crashes nearly nine times greater than a driver at zero BAC. The risk for such a driver with BAC between 0.10 and 0.14 percent is forty times as high as without alcohol, and for a driver with 0.15 percent or more, six hundred times as high. Moreover, "when plausible assumptions were made about the BAC distributions of other participants in multiple-vehicle crashes (whose actual BAC is often unknown), the relative risks based on the maximum BAC of the crash participants were nearly as high as those estimated in single vehicle crashes" (Zador, 1989: i).

These estimates might be taken to suggest that drivers in the lower BAC categories could be ignored because they are much less dangerous than those with higher BACs. However, because there are so many more drivers, driving many more miles, in the low than in the high categories, low-BAC drivers are also found to contribute to total casualties.

The bulk of alcohol-related crash deaths—and the greatest need for social interventions—lies among drivers with highly elevated BACs. For example, in 1989, 31.7 percent of drivers involved in fatal crashes were found when tested to have consumed alcohol. Most—24.2 percent—had BACs above 0.10 percent (National Highway Traffic Safety Administration, 1991). However, the fact that an important segment of fatality-involved impaired drivers nonetheless had low to moderate BACS should not be forgotten. Moreover, drivers with modest BACs appear to form a large fraction of those in crashes resulting in injuries and particularly of those involving property damage (Jones and Joscelyn, 1978: 27). The policy implication of these observations is not the need to stress measures aimed at the less extreme group, but rather to welcome interventions that include these drivers as well as the more impaired. Put otherwise, the fact that a drunk driving countermeasure impinges on moderate drinkers is not a reason to reject it, but rather an additional reason to adopt it.

If this definition of the problem is accepted, then the dominant and accepted typification of drunk driving—the "killer drunk" image—is misleading. Gusfield (1981: 112) identifies the typification in a court decision of 1921, which he summarizes as follows: "The drinking driver is a serious malfeasant; he is not the average citizen, the 'natural man' who sometimes speeds, makes a left turn against a prohibiting sign, or otherwise acts in the foolish or perverse manner of you and me. . . . [T]he driver who enters traffic under the influence of alcohol is a sinner against others." In later passages Gusfield (1981: 153) elaborates the contents of this typification:

21

The first [aspect of the drinking-driver's villainy] is the *antisocial character of drinking-driving*.... To drive after drinking is ... to show disregard for others—to place self-indulgence above orderly conduct toward others. It takes risks not only with self but with "society." Every drinking-driver is the "killer-drunk."

A second aspect of the drinking-driver's villainy is his *responsibility for his actions*. . . . A person in command and control of his behavior, he is liable for the crime committed. . . .

The third aspect of the drinking-driver's villainy is his *status as a deviant—morally and factually*. His crime is not the minor one of traffic offense.

A contemporary statement embodying this typification can be found in Alan Dershowitz's syndicated newspaper column for September 3, 1990: "The most serious crime in America is not drug use, or rape or armed robbery. It is drunken driving. And the most dangerous criminals are not drug addicts, organized criminals, or professional burglars [but, rather, impaired drivers]." Dershowitz subsequently raises questions about the typification by describing the villains as young and middle-class and by indicating that some are women. However, association of drunk driving with violent crimes like rape and robbery, and of drunk drivers with vicious people like professional criminals, characterizes past and present approaches to drunk driving in America. This image is highly stereotyped and greatly oversimplifies a complex and tragic situation.

Perhaps the most fundamental difference between my definition of drunk driving and drunk driving as generally typified lies in the fact that my definition covers situations in which criminal law does not apply—where the behavior falls short of legal standards of "drunkenness" or "intoxication" or where, in addition, the driver's BAC does not exceed the legal limit—and which are therefore literally *not* crimes. My definition implies that there is no qualitative distinction between use and abuse of alcohol in association with driving. It focuses on the relative dangerousness of the behavior rather than the deviance and irresponsibility of the drunk driver. Many people who put themselves and others at significantly elevated risk of serious crashes because they drive while impaired by alcohol cannot be regarded as deviant, and their moral responsibility is obscured because their behavior conforms to prevailing expectations concerning the conditions of sociable interaction. Others, although deviant according to general social norms and illegal to boot, may be viewed as conforming to the norms of more restricted communities, such as some college fraternities. In noting this, I am not arguing for their toleration, but rather for understanding so that prevention can intelligently be planned.

The extent of drunk driving

The banality or ordinariness of drunk driving is hinted at by the fact that arrests, rare as they may be in relation to acts of drunk driving, number more than a million in the United States every year. An analysis of records in Minnesota, where the data are of good quality, has found that 8 percent of all licensed drivers had one or more drunk driving violations on their record (Rodgers, 1990). New Mexico officials say, in a private communication, that drunk driving convictions appear on the records of 14 percent of drivers in that state.

Although these figures may serve to alarm, they do not give a very useful idea of the magnitude of the problem in terms of numbers of impaired trips experienced in a month or a year or numbers of impaired miles driven. This is needed for the purpose, among others, of appraising the relative dangerousness of impaired driving through putting the figures of alcohol-related crash deaths and injuries into the context of the amount of exposure. It is also needed in order to form realistic goals and expectations of results for countermeasure programs.

There are three common sources of such information. These are, first, traditional telephone or in-person surveys to elicit self-reports of behavior; second, breath tests of drivers sampled from the highway; and, third, extrapolations from blood tests of drivers in fatal crashes.

Traditional survey data

There is a large literature based on self-reports of drunk driving. The data are obtained from public opinion surveys, often carried out by telephone. A general problem with this literature is that self-reported behavior may well differ from actual behavior, especially when the behavior to be reported is, like drunk driving or even alcohol consumption, believed to be not fully countenanced by society. In this situation, survey results tend to yield underestimates of the extent of the undesirable behavior. The following findings must be interpreted in light of this caution.

Perhaps surprisingly, then, the proportions of respondents admitting to having ever driven while impaired or intoxicated can be quite high. For example, the *Wall Street Journal* (1983) reported a Gallup poll in which 80 percent of business executives (85 percent of those under age fifty) said they had driven while drunk. The same admission was made by 46 percent of men in a sample drawn from the general public.

If large proportions of businessmen admit to driving after drinking, it is not surprising to find that their children follow suit. A study of 192 students in middle-class urban and suburban schools in the Seattle area found 79 percent admitting to drinking alcohol, and of those who drank, 58 percent admitted to driving after drinking, at least occasionally. The sample of sixteen- to nineteen-year-olds who had been driving for at least six months and had *no* drunk driving citations nonetheless produced reports of 404 incidents of driving after consuming alcohol or other drugs (Farrow, 1987). The investigator has stated, "Young drivers appeared to drink in a variety of environments, with particularly high consumption taking place at the homes of friends, in public places, parks, and an automobile. Given the high mobility of this group of drivers, it appears that a significant amount of driving is done under the influence of alcohol or marijuana" (Farrow, 1985: 372).

More than half of male and a third of female first-year students sampled from Boston-area colleges said they had driven after drinking in the past year, despite the fact that all were under the legal minimum drinking age (Wechsler and Isaac, 1991). What is more, nearly one young man in five in this sample admitted to driving after having consumed five or more drinks.

The national Health Interview Survey (Williams, DuFour, and Bertolucci, 1986), based on field data from 1985, found admissions of drunk driving to be common, if not as universal as in the polls reported above. Asked whether in the past year they had driven one or more times when they had had too much to drink, 23 percent of the male respondents and 10 percent of the female responded positively.

A repeated Roper poll for the All-Industry Research Advisory Council found 37 percent of a national sample in 1985 and 28 percent in 1988 admitting to driving after consuming alcohol (*New York Times*, 1988). The poll apparently did not inquire, however, how much alcohol was consumed before driving.

In Minnesota, a state noted for aggressive anti-drunk-driving measures, a poll of drivers conducted in 1985 found 71 percent admitting to having driven within two hours of consuming alcohol at some point in the previous year, and 37 percent admitting to having driven when they thought they were over the legal limit. Moreover, 28 percent said they were likely to drive while intoxicated at some point in the future (Cleary, Shapiro, and Williams, 1986). The same figure, 28 percent, was reported among the results of a face-to-face interview survey in Oklahoma City in 1985 concerning expectations of driving "while under the influence of a moderate amount of alcohol" (Grasmick and Bursik, 1990).

The percentages reported in these examples must be appreciated in light of the fact that about a third of the general public (but apparently far fewer business executives) are nondrinkers. If the questions were limited to people who do drink, some of the proportions would be higher. Underestimation of drunk driving as defined here is rendered more likely when questions are phrased in terms of driving "when you had too much to drink" or "when you had too much to drive safely," because people's ideas about "too much" may be limited to gross intoxication. Moreover, drunk driving's negative publicity during the past decade is likely to have reduced the proportion of people willing to admit to it, so that true figures are most likely higher than those obtained in the surveys. Even when not adjusted for these potential biases, public opinion polls support a picture of drunk driving as common and conventional, rather than extreme and deviant. They also suggest that drunk driving may be more common among high-status people such as business executives than among the public in general.

Roadside surveys

The second approach to estimating the size of the drunk-driving problem relies on breath-testing of drivers from the population on the highway. Such roadside surveys are expensive. Moreover, the use of police officers to stop cars and divert them off the road for questioning is imperative, yet a growing concern among administrators over exposure to new sources of legal liability has reduced the willingness of many police departments to cooperate with drunk driving surveys. Roadside surveys are therefore not numerous, but they are especially valuable because they directly measure the BACs of drivers on the road.

Most such surveys have been limited to individual communities or, at best, to states (see, for example, Ross and Voas, 1989; Palmer and Tix, 1985). Fortunately, recent national data are available from a 1985 survey of drivers funded by the Insurance Institute for Highway Safety (Lund and Wolfe, 1991). Like most roadside surveys, this one concentrated on the days of the week and times of day when drunk driving is most likely to occur, in particular Fridays and Saturdays from 9 P.M. until 3 A.M. the next morning. The researchers were able to obtain breath tests for 92 percent of the drivers, and summary statistics were weighted to correct for possible refusal bias. A total of 8.4 percent of the drivers were judged to have BACs equal to or greater than 0.05 percent. The fact that on a given weekend night, 1 out of 12 drivers had impairing concentrations of alcohol in their blood indicates that drunk driving in this broad sense is a fairly common experience for Americans. However, a survey based on similar methods performed in 1973 had found evidence of impairment in 13.7 percent of drivers, a much higher fraction, suggesting that a reduction in drunk driving occurred during the intervening years, even if the problem still seems relatively widespread.

A weakness of roadside surveys is that, in the United States at least, participation is voluntary. Since drunk drivers are a minority of those stopped and may be more likely than most drivers to refuse to cooperate in surveys, the reported data probably underestimate the amount of drunk driving. Comparison of responses between years is hazardous because during the interval willingness to admit the behavior may have changed. Roadside survey responses should be regarded as providing an estimate of the lower limit of the true proportion of impaired drivers.

Crash-fatality data

The third approach to estimating the size of the drunk-driving problem involves studies of drivers in fatal crashes. These form a small but important fraction of drunk drivers. Data on fatal crashes appear to be more complete and reliable than those on other kinds of crashes, and they are easily available to researchers and policy makers through the federal Fatal Accident Reporting System (FARS) data bank.

The relationship between conditions in fatal crashes and those among drivers in general may not be constant, and proper use of this data base must respect its limitations. Especially important is the matter of incomplete testing. Because tests for alcohol are most frequently taken from those suspected of being under the influence, jurisdictions with small testing fractions tend to find high proportions of positive results (Ostrom et al., 1991); similar jurisdictions with large fractions of tested drivers find lower proportions of positive results.

For various reasons it is not possible to obtain useful data on 100 percent of drivers in serious crashes. One reason is the occasional lengthy delay between a crash and the opportunity to test the driver, during which time alcohol becomes metabolized and disappears from the body if the driver is still living. Testing rates of 80 percent or more are considered acceptable and are attained by approximately half the states as of this writing. The FARS system offers statistical formulas to adjust estimates for underreporting that may remain. Prior to 1984, national estimates prepared by the FARS staff were based on data provided by the fifteen states with the most complete reporting; since then, the estimates have been based on data from all states, adjusted by the formulas to take underreporting into account.

These data support the impression that drunk driving is common in America. That they are drawn from incidents involving violent death underscores the devastating potential of alcohol impairment. In recent years, the proportion of drivers in fatal crashes found positive for alcohol (in any detectable amount) has been about a third, most of these having BACs of at least 0.10 percent (National Highway Traffic Safety Administration, 1989; Fell and Nash, 1989). In 1989, 37 percent of all drivers who were themselves fatally injured had BACs exceeding 0.10 percent (National Center for Statistics and Analysis, 1990). FARS data are made available annually, and changes and trends in this data base can confirm impressions based on other, broader but less reliable data. For instance, the impression of a reduction in drunk driving in America is supported in FARS data as well as in roadside surveys of drivers in general.

Summary

In sum, all major methods of estimating drunk driving support the conclusion that it is widespread in American society. A reasonable general estimate based on a broad review is given by Nichols (1990: 45–46). He estimates that approximately 20 percent of American drivers, or 33 million persons, drive while illegally impaired at least once per year. It is likely that the figure would be considerably higher if those driving legally but impaired were added. Such estimates point to the commonplace and conventional nature of drunk driving in America, explainable in large part by our distinctive institutions of transportation and leisure.

Causes of drunk driving in America

Social problems have social causes. Like other social problems, drunk driving is a product of established ways of doing things, of accepted and valued institutions. The problems can be seen as the undesired dark side of arrangements that from other viewpoints strike us as good and desirable. Thus, theft can be seen as a predictable consequence of the acceptance and valuing of material goods in America, along with a democratic egalitarianism concerning standards for ownership and use. Abortion may be the price of freedom of affection and sexuality in a society that insists on moralistic constraints on education and communications about sexual behavior. Political corruption may be an understandable product of penurious governmental stipends and an electoral process that requires enormous resources. Similarly, drunk driving is a product of America's commitments to alcohol as a drug of recreation and hospitality and to the automobile as the near-exclusive means of transportation.

Commitment to the use of alcohol

Alcohol as an organic chemical substance is identical throughout the world. Alcohol as a consumer commodity, however, differs widely from society to society. Klaus Mäkelä (1983) posits three meanings or varieties of use that, he argues, are present in all societies but are more or less prominent depending on place and time. These are nutritional use, medical use, and intoxicant use. Medical use, the rarest, accounts for the fact that in many countries experiencing prohibition, exceptions were made for patent medicines. In the United States, pillars of the Woman's Christian Temperance Union used tonics that frequently contained not only alcohol, but narcotics as well. Alcohol and other drugs when used as medicines often escape being labeled as problematic, even in societies suspicious of mind-altering substances, because their perceived therapeutic potential distracts attention from their intoxicant potential. In a parallel manner, societies like those of Italy and France stress the role of alcoholic beverages, especially wine, as food. Again the intoxicant role is deemphasized, this time in favor of the nutritional role. In contrast, people in countries such as Russia, Finland, Sweden, Norway, and Iceland emphasize the intoxicant aspect of alcohol and view its proper use as that of producing inebriation.

The dominant, though not exclusive, American definition of alcohol strikes me as involving yet a different image—that of social lubricant. Alcohol belongs in leisure situations because it stimulates friendly, relaxed interaction. Used this way, it is part of the good life. Close friends meet at the bar over drinks. Good hosts set their guests at ease by offering a drink and ensuring that a generous supply of alcohol is available throughout the social occasion.

These differences may be illustrated with an anecdote. On my first visit to Finland I had the pleasure of lunching with Inkeri Anttila, a criminologist who at that time was serving as the country's minister of justice. I ordered a bottle of beer to drink with lunch. Dr. Anttila was amused: "Most people in this country would say that you are wasting your money. You will drink that expensive beer with lunch and not feel a thing!" she said. "Instead, you should save your lunch money for Saturday night and then order seven beers. That way, you will feel them, which is what the beer is for!" By consuming a small dose of alcohol with a meal, an accepted practice for a Frenchman or a middle-class American, I was abusing the substance by Finnish standards.

If drinking for the purpose of becoming intoxicated knows nearly no bounds other than stupor—more high is better than less—the other uses of alcohol contain implicit limits on consumption. Medicine should be taken in the proper amount to cure the symptom. Although too small a dose may fail to provide the desired relief, too much may produce undesirable side effects. When alcohol is consumed as food, there are again limits. One should eat and drink to satiation, not to excess. Eating when one is hungry is pleasant, but being overfed is not. Similarly, when alcohol is a social lubricant, it loses its main purpose if taken to excess. Drunkenness is not, in the dominant American view, a necessarily desirable state. Excessive consumption leads to disorder and violence, rather than sociability. The normative drinker should ordinarily consume alcohol in moderation.

The American view of alcohol, then, contains both inducements ("Beer belongs") and cautions ("Know when to say when") as influences on consumption. Commercial advertising and marketing strategies generally attempt to renew and reinforce the inducements, while laws and regulations generally support the cautions. The resultant pattern is described in a report by the National Research Council of the National Academy of Sciences:

Approximately one-third of the adult population is abstinent. Another third averages no more (most average less) than 3 drinks per week and seldom gets drunk. The next fifth or so of the population averages 3 drinks or more a day and gets drunk more than once a week. The remaining 1–5 percent of the population (a more exact percentage is difficult to ascertain) averages 10 drinks or more per day and spends most days of the year above the level of 8 drinks. [Moore and Gerstein, 1981: 32–33]

A more recent report from the National Institute on Alcohol Abuse and Alcoholism (U.S. Department of Health and Human Services, 1990: 2), based on survey data from 1985, presents a similar picture: 34 percent of the population declared themselves nondrinkers, 56 percent were "nondependent, nonproblem," or "social," drinkers, and 10 percent were problem drinkers, about half of them alcohol dependent.

Briefly, most Americans are drinkers; total abstention might be termed deviant behavior. Among those who drink, most drink moderately in terms of total consumption, but consumption tends to be concentrated (for instance, at night and on weekends), producing higher BACs on occasion than would dispersed consumption (such as occurs in France and Italy) of the same amount of alcohol.

There are subgroups in American society for whom alcohol has still other meanings, including its being the measure of manhood and masculinity. These subgroups, disproportionately found among young people and, according to some evidence, blacks and Hispanics, encourage and tolerate a greater consumption of alcohol than does the general consensus (e.g., National Institute on Alcohol Abuse and Alcoholism, 1985; Wechsler and Isaac, 1991; Ross et al., 1991). Moreover, membership in these subgroups is likely to foster concentrated, or binge, drinking, which is disproportionately associated with alcohol-related problems (Moore and Gerstein, 1981).

Norms specifying frequent and heavy use of alcohol are also found among people who, through disease or other processes, have developed a life-style centered around drinking. Whether it is profitable to call them alcoholics or problem drinkers or—as urged by Fingarette

(1988)—merely heavy drinkers, the routine consumption of prodigious amounts of alcohol is common and expected in their social circles (Wiseman, 1979). To the extent that such individuals drive, they pose extraordinary risks of serious injury and death to themselves and others.

The distribution of alcohol problems, including drunk driving, reflects both the consumption patterns and the size of each subgroup. Drinking that conforms to general norms, which set limits on occasions and amount of alcohol consumed, can easily lead to BACs that significantly elevate the risk of serious crashes. Drinking that conforms to the norms of heavier-drinking subgroups produces much greater risks, although the contribution of the subgroups to the total drunk driving problem is limited by their numbers. As stated in the National Research Council report,

> While chronic drinkers with high consumption both cause and suffer more than their numerical share of the adverse consequences of drinking, their share of alcohol problems is still only a fraction—typically less than half—of the total. Alcohol problems occur *throughout* the drinking population. They occur at lower rates but among much greater numbers as one moves from the heaviest to more moderate drinkers. [Moore and Gerstein, 1981: 44]

The American commitment to alcohol is bolstered by the nation's deeply rooted alcoholic beverage industry. The wholesale value of alcoholic beverages produced in the United States has amounted to more than $20 billion annually in recent years (U.S. Department of Commerce, 1989). Moreover, production is just one part of the industry, which also includes wholesaling, distribution, and retailing. The retail branch makes the beverage industry an integral part of nearly every community in the nation. The brewing segment alone (which accounts for slightly more than half of the industry's sales) used over a million retail outlets to sell products valued at $43 billion at retail in 1987. It directly provided about 900,000 jobs, paying more than $10 billion in wages. The industry claims that through the "multiplier effect" an additional 1.2 million jobs and more than $20 billion in wages were generated. On this basis, beer can be said to have made economic contributions in excess of $1 billion in thirty states in 1987 (Barsby and Associates, 1988).

The alcoholic beverage industry is also intimately involved with the nation's media. The following figures were mentioned in a letter of June 1990 to various congressmen from Harold Shoup, representing a group of advertising, alcohol, and media executives. In 1988, beer and wine advertising accounted for 4.6 percent of all television advertising, 7.1 percent of radio advertising, 3.6 percent of magazine advertising, 1.7 percent of newspaper advertising, and 5.6 percent of outdoor advertising. Were these expenditures to decline, for example, because of unwillingness of sponsors to accept health warning labels on their advertising, the consequences predicted include reduced income and lost jobs in the media and reduced entertainment and sports programming for the public. The message of much of this alcohol advertising is that drinking is not only normal, but is a vital and valuable component of the American life-style, especially for men (see Postman et al., 1987).

Society's commitment to alcohol is further promoted by the alcoholic beverage industry's involvement in politics, through lobbying organizations and political contributions. Between 1985 and 1988, the industry contributed more than $4 million to congressional campaigns (Center for Science in the Public Interest, 1989). Over three-quarters of members of the 100th Congress received honoraria or Political Action Committee (PAC) contributions from the alcohol industry.

In summary, American society has institutionalized the use of alcoholic beverages, and most Americans participate in this use. Alcohol is regarded primarily as a social lubricant, implying the legitimacy of its use on occasions of sociable leisure as well as normative constraints on the amounts consumed. In some circles, norms of heavier and more concentrated drinking prevail, and for a small minority of people, alcohol has become a central life activity with virtually no limits to appropriate drinking.

Conformity to general norms for the use of alcohol in America is likely to lead to BACs which, when present in drivers, significantly increase the risk of a serious crash. Socially acceptable drinking, perhaps roughly corresponding to that of the middle third and part of the next 20 percent of the National Academy of Science's model, is easily capable of doubling and tripling the risk of a fatal crash. Furthermore, higher BACs (and therefore magnified chances of serious crashes) are normatively prescribed in specific subgroups in American society, especially among young men and among people of all ages who have developed life-styles centered on heavy drinking. Members of these groups are disproportionately hazardous while on the road, and the extreme magnification of crash risk among them situates them at the heart of the fatality issue. However, their centrality to the drunk driving problem should not obscure the contribution of the much larger population that drinks more conventionally, with elevation of crash risk nonetheless. The commitment to alcohol in all strata of American society is encouraged by the existence of strong, pervasive vested interests, including producers, distributors, and retailers of beverages.

Commitment to the use of automobiles

The United States has the most lavish supply of automobiles in the entire world. About a third of all registered automobiles are to be found in this country. Across the whole world there are about 10 people per motor vehicle, whereas in the United States the ratio is 1.4 to 1 (Motor Vehicle Manufacturers Association [MVMA], 1989: 36–37). In 1983, fewer than 14 percent of American households lacked cars; about a third had two cars, and nearly one in five had three or more cars (MVMA, 1989: 46).

Americans are not only well provided with automobiles; most are nearly totally dependent on them. In 1983, private motor vehicles were used for 82 percent of all trips for any purpose. They were involved in 80 percent of trips for family and personal business, such as shopping, going to school and church, and obtaining medical and dental care; 84 percent of trips for social and recreational purposes; and 87 percent of trips between home and work. In contrast, public transportation by bus, streetcar, subway, train, airplane, taxi, and elevated train combined was used for just 2.5 percent of trips overall; 2 percent of trips for family and personal business, 1 percent of trips for social and recreational purposes, and 5 percent of trips between home and work (MVMA, 1989: 50–51). Despite criticism of the automobile's massive consumption of resources, its contribution to environmental pollution, and its annual toll of lives, injuries, and ruined property (e.g., Schneider, 1971; Slovenko, 1983), private vehicle ownership and mileage continue to grow, to the point that in many communities rival transportation systems have virtually disappeared. Assuming near-universal automobile ownership, developers of the American landscape have created a fabric of low-density housing and dispersed destinations which can be efficiently served only by a fleet of private automobiles. In terms of comfort, convenience, and internalized costs, the automobile is triumphant. The car-less person is a social cripple: "A paradox of growing automobility is that persons without cars become less mobile as a large portion of society begins to travel predominantly by car, partly because transit options are cut back as riders switch to driving and partly because urban areas and essential travel destinations tend to spread out as auto use becomes more universal" (Altshuler et al., 1984: 75). Moreover, as is evident in voluminous popular literature, the automobile is not mere transportation. The car offers privacy, status, and freedom itself. For these reasons, Americans demand and are permitted near-universal participation in driving. In 1989, 165 million people, more than 85 percent of the population sixteen years of age or older, were licensed to drive. Among younger men, licensure is practically universal. Such a proportion of drivers can be achieved only with extremely liberal criteria for participation in the pool. Numerous drivers must be subnormal in intelligence, legally blind, physically and emotionally immature, senile, and alcoholic, reflecting the proportions of such people in the general population. The car is the key to the most meaningful forms of American citizenship, and in practice we are loath to deny its privileges to anyone who has not repeatedly demonstrated gross abuses of the public trust.

This commitment, like that to alcohol, is supported by potent commercial and industrial interests. The business of manufacturing motor vehicles and equipment is one of the country's largest: in 1986, there were nearly four thousand domestic manufacturing facilities, employing three-quarters of a million workers, with a payroll of $36 billion. Although the industry bulks largest in Michigan, significant numbers of facilities can be found in nearly all states: payrolls in Ohio, Indiana, Missouri, New York, and Wisconsin as well as Michigan each exceed a billion dollars annually. Total employment related to building, selling, driving, maintaining, and otherwise providing for motor vehicles amounts to more than 12 million jobs, or nearly 15 percent of U.S. employment (MVMA, 1989: 66–68).

These facts support the characterization of America as committed to the private automobile. In conjunction with the commitment to the use of alcohol, documented above, widespread engaging in drinking and driving, driving impaired by alcohol, and drunk driving in both broad and narrow senses is preordained. This does not mean that the problem is intractable, but that major and lasting reductions will necessitate changes in basic social institutions. Such changes can be expected to be resisted initially by large fractions of the public, and the status quo will be defended by the powerful economic interests vested in current institutional arrangements. However, to the extent that policy makers and citizens understand the links between institutions and social problems, there are grounds for hope that changes can be made.

The consequences of drunk driving

Appreciating the consequences of drunk driving involves coping with a paradox. On the one hand, drunk driving greatly increases the risk of a crash, especially a fatal one. On the other hand, the likelihood of a crash fatality on any given trip—even an alcohol-impaired one—remains extremely low. Our lavish and almost exclusive use of automobiles for travel testifies to our perception that the likelihood of any contemplated trip being interrupted by a serious crash is negligible. Although the media offer news of serious crashes almost daily, we act as though the probability of our personal involvement were, to all intents, zero. In everyday experience, people who tremble with fright when thinking about flying on a scheduled airline can blithely get behind the wheel of a car for a journey that is objectively far more dangerous (but perhaps only for long trips—see the argument of Evans, Frick, and Schwing, 1990, and the comment by Sivak, Weintraub, and Flannagan, 1991). A different, more fearful view of automobile crash risk might be greatly upsetting to the American life-style.

Some statistics can be read to support the public impression of near perfect safety for automobile occupants. The mileage-based crash death rate, which includes the deaths of bicyclists, motorcyclists, and pedestrians in addition to those of automobile drivers and passengers, has been declining with few reversals for several decades and now is in the neighborhood of 2 per 100 million vehicle miles traveled. The risk of dying in the course of a five-mile journey by car can thus be estimated at about 1 in 10 million, which from most viewpoints would be considered truly negligible. Most important, a doubling or even a hundredfold increase in this probability also produces an apparently negligible risk. As we learned in school, anything multiplied by "zero" is equal to zero. Therefore, from one viewpoint, the harmfulness of drunk driving fails to be evident or impressive.

The other side of the paradox is visible through different statistics, those that take account of the enormous numbers of miles driven in America. Motor vehicle travel in this country amounts to close to 2 trillion miles annually. Considering this exposure, the highly unlikely possibility of a mishap when confronting the individual trip becomes in the aggregate an awful certainty. The American highway transportation system regularly and predictably produces forty thousand or more fatalities each year. The declining death rate mentioned above fails to staunch the loss because it is compensated for by rising mileage, which increases the exposure.

Slightly less than half of these deaths occur in crashes in which some measurable amount of alcohol is present (National Highway Traffic Safety Administration, 1989; 1991; National Center for Statistics and Analysis, 1990). As I have cautioned previously, not all of these can be said to have been caused by drunk driving. In some cases, the only alcohol present was in the body of a person other than a driver, such as a pedestrian or a bicyclist. In others, the driver's BAC may have been only trivially elevated, in a range where little increment in crash risk has been demonstrated. Even in those crashes involving a highly impaired driver, causation and responsibility might lie elsewhere.

The distinction between causation and association or correlation is not always respected in policy discussions. For example, former president Ronald Reagan, in his introduction to the Final Report of the Presidential Commission on Drunk Driving (1983), stated, "Over the past ten years, 250,000 Americans have died in accidents caused (*sic*) by drunk driving, and millions have been maimed or crippled." In making this erroneous statement, the president was misled by his commission, which on page 1 of the body of its report asserted, "At least 50 percent of all highway deaths involve the irresponsible use of alcohol." Had President Reagan and the commission been correct, all the fatal crashes in which any alcohol was found would have been caused by drunk driving. This is clearly implausible. For example, as Evans (1991) notes, it is possible that caffeine from coffee was present in even more of the crash casualties, yet if that were shown, few people would conclude that it was an important causal factor. It is in part alcohol's ambivalent social reputation that seems to permit the logical leaps noted here.

Estimating the proportion of fatalities in which alcohol is a causal factor is a difficult task. One might attempt it by looking at each case individually. Although this could eliminate obvious exceptions, such as the hypotheticals mentioned in the previous paragraph, few if any crashes involving drivers with positive BACs could, from data typically available, be confidently either ascribed to alcohol or excluded from the possibility that alcohol had a causal role. A much better approach compares the distributions of BACs among crash-involved drivers and control drivers not involved in crashes and selected from times and places similar to the crash-involved. To the extent that alcohol is disproportionately present among the crash-involved it is possible to compute how many crashes might have been avoided if all drivers had consumed no alcohol. Such an analysis was performed by David Reed for the National Research Council (Moore and Gerstein, 1981: 336–87), based largely on a reanalysis of Vermont fatality and control data from 1967–68. Reed concluded that about half of all alcohol-related fatal crashes—and therefore about a quarter of total fatal crashes—would have been avoided if all drivers had BACs of zero. This is much less than the numbers mentioned by President Reagan, his Commission on Drunk Driving, and most other participants in policy discussion of the past decade, but it accords rather well with a previous estimate by Richard Zylman (1974), based on more limited data. More recent work by Evans (1990; 1991) based on death statistics in twenty-six states claims a larger causal role for alcohol in highway crashes. However, the presence of various dubious or contestable assumptions in the calculations, and the contrast of this work with the balance of the literature, militate against quickly abandoning the latter in favor of Evans's estimates.

The proportion of deaths meaningfully caused by alcohol—those that would be avoided were alcohol not present—provides a target, in the sense of an ideal outer limit rather than a practical goal, for saving lives with countermeasures directed at drunk driving. The target appears to be lower than that suggested in many sources, both official and unofficial. For instance, it appears unrealistic to think that "[i]f the [drunk-driving] problem is properly managed by federal, state and local governments . . . instead of a yearly [highway] death toll of 25,000 killed and 650,000 injured, at least half that number could be spared" (Golden, 1983: 11).

In saying that deaths due to drunk driving (and the possible value of countermeasures) may be overestimated I do not mean to trivialize the drunk driving problem or demean the importance of policies aimed at controlling it. Alcohol is the largest single specifiable cause of crash deaths, and the reduction of its presence on the road is a major life-saving opportunity. On the basis of his rather conservative estimate of alcohol's causal role in crashes, Reed saw "maximum achievable savings in 1977 of 11,700 deaths, 156,000 to 300,000 disabling injuries, and $963 million in property damage" (Moore and Gerstein, 1981: 340). These are hardly trivial sums! Moreover, as Reed also indicates, deaths in crashes typically occur among a younger age group than is involved in deaths from other major causes, resulting in the loss of a higher number of potential years of life than with most other causes of death. Reducing drunk driving would reduce not only deaths, but also injuries and property damage. If the economic costs of injuries and property damage were even half the presidential commission estimate of $21 to $25 billion, there would be much benefit beyond lifesaving to reward measures that successfully reduce drunk driving.

The drunk driving problem today

Social problems, in the political sense discussed here, often lose their saliency and disappear from political consciousness even when there is no evidence of changes in fundamental conditions (Jolly and Mills, 1984). The soldiers in President Lyndon Johnson's War on Poverty, for example, were never able to declare victory, but they and the poverty problem faded away with little public notice or concern (Katz, 1989). Poverty has little chance of being named a major problem on the political agenda of the 1990s, in contrast to crime or drugs, for example. However, unlike the poverty problem, drunk driving appears to remain a viable concern after a decade of prominence. Even though media attention to drunk driving and the growth of victims' organizations like Mothers Against Drunk Driving (MADD) peaked in the mid–1980s (McCarthy, Wolfson, and Harvey, 1987), a citizen activist was able in 1988 to obtain a virtually unanimous Concurrent Resolution of the U.S. House and Senate (H. Con. Res. 276, March 31, 1988) requesting that the surgeon general declare a national crisis in the matter of drunk driving. (The surgeon general responded to this call by convening a workshop of national experts, whose report in 1989 helped launch drunk driving as a social problem into the next decade.)

Jolly and Mills point out that drunk driving resembles problems that tend to cycle out of existence, in that the majority of people do not suffer from the problem but rather benefit from the conditions (extensive leisure drinking and extensive driving) that create it, and that the problem is not inherently exciting over the long term. However, it differs in that drunk driving, at least according to the ruling typification, involves a simple, obvious injustice perpetrated on an innocent victim and also in that drinking drivers form an easily targeted scapegoat that can be attacked without fear of retaliation or the antagonizing of a large proportion of the population. Jolly and Mills point out that these differences may prolong the life of the problem. To their credit, they also note that the perceived differences are rooted in "rather naive notions" of the problem: "As people come to realize that the roots of the problem are deep and entangled with longstanding social patterns of drinking and of driving, then the enthusiasm for simple solutions of stricter enforcement and adjudication will likely wane and with it much of the attention the issue has received" (1984: 7–8).

If *crisis* remains an acceptable label for the drunk-driving problem as a political matter, data from the field suggest that occasions of impaired driving have been declining. The best evidence concerning changes in the BACs of drivers on the highways appears in the contrast between the results of the survey sponsored by the Insurance Institute for Highway Safety in 1986 (Lund and Wolfe, 1991) and the similar survey sponsored by the National Highway Traffic Safety Administration in 1973 (Wolfe, 1973). Although changes in the street layout and traffic patterns in cities, difficulties in obtaining cooperation from police departments, and differences in the testing instruments of the two surveys must be kept in mind, the sophisticated methodology used statistical corrections for possible biases such as those due to refusals and large samples to increase the precision of estimates. Comparison of the results of the two surveys showed a considerable reduction in BACs of drivers on weekend nights. For example, BACs equal to or exceeding 0.10 percent were found in 5.1 percent of the sample in 1973, but only in 3.2 percent in 1986. BACs equal to at least 0.05 percent were found in 13.7 percent of drivers in the earlier survey, but only in 8.4 percent in the more recent survey. Looking at subgroups in the population, the comparison found that the declines were quite general, for example, between the sexes and among geographical regions. Exceptions to the general finding did occur for some groups; for instance, blacks and Hispanics did not show significant declines in the proportion of drivers with high BACs. However, only tentative conclusions about minority drivers are warranted because of their small numbers in both surveys.

The picture of declining proportions of alcohol-impaired drivers is confirmed by information on drivers in fatal crashes from the FARS data bank. The proportion of fatally injured drivers with BACs of at least 0.10 percent decreased fairly regularly between 1980, when it was 46 percent, and 1985, when it was 39 percent, and irregularly since that time to the figure of 37 percent in 1989 (National Center for Statistics and Analysis, 1990). The percentage of drivers in fatal crashes with BACs of 0.10 percent and more fell from 30 in 1982 to 25 in 1987 (Fell and Nash, 1989). Among teenagers, the decline was from 29 percent to 19 percent, a reduction of fully a third. Although similar declines were noted in most groups, there were some exceptions, including drivers aged twenty- five to thirty-four and motorcyclists, and the declines were more modest in late-night and single-vehicle crashes, in which the drunk-driving problem is most deeply ingrained. This might suggest that the most problematic of drinking drivers were changing the least, but the fraction of FARS drivers with extraordinarily high BACs (equaling or exceeding 0.20 percent) declined the most, while that with BACs under 0.10 percent was unchanged, in keeping with the view that the most impaired drunk drivers changed the most.

Some of this moderation would have been expected even in the absence of any deliberate social policy to combat drunk driving because of changes in overall alcohol consumption in the country—perhaps part of a growing health consciousness—and a reduction in the numbers of people in the demographic group with the highest drunk driving involvement, young people under age twenty-four. However, the reductions seem too great to be totally explained by these factors, and absent other plausible rival explanations it is reasonable to conclude that some part of the change noted occurred in response to policy interventions (Williams, 1991).

The remainder of this book surveys the American experience with attempts to control drunk driving and its tragic consequences of deaths and injuries. It will suggest what is working among the policies that are currently being applied, which may account for some of the favorable evolution in statistics noted here. In so doing it will also note policies that seem to be ineffective or inefficient, which should be either modified or abandoned in favor of more promising ones. It will survey the opportunities available for making further progress, including those with promise based on experience, along with promising interventions that have not yet been tried or sufficiently evaluated. The book is not intended to dismiss all that has been done so far in the way of policy to reduce drunk driving. Rather, I intend to acknowledge past successes, urging their retention and strengthening, while directing attention to new measures as well. The task is not just one of deletions, but also of substitutions and of additions to the armory of countermeasures to drunk driving.

Law and Criminal Justice

"The cornerstone of all efforts to reduce the problem of alcohol- impaired driving is state laws making driving with high BACs illegal" (Williams, 1989: 3). This is the situation even though such laws do not deal with the fundamental causes of drunk driving as diagnosed here. Criminal justice interventions attempt to overcome social incentives to drunk driving by attaching a threat of punishment to the dangerous behavior sufficient to dissuade the potential drunk driver from carrying out his intentions. The primary mechanism involved is that of general deterrence, a principle that predicts effects on behavior in proportion to the perceived severity, certainty, and swiftness of the legal threat. This chapter reviews the history of drunk driving law. It analyzes the place of deterrence among the functions of the criminal law and evaluates the extent and means by which drunk driving laws are able to accomplish the function of deterrence.

Drunk driving law in America

The attempt to deal criminally with drunk driving has characterized American policy since the dawn of the automotive age. Even before World War I, New York and California adopted laws prohibiting impaired driving and stipulating punishments that included jail terms and license suspension. By 1924, Connecticut was jailing more than two hundred drivers per year for the offense (Voas and Lacey, 1989: 137).

The early laws, which I have called classical (Ross, 1982), proved difficult to apply because they required proof of a state of "drunk" driving,

3

driving "under the influence of alcohol" (DUI), or driving "while impaired by alcohol" (DWI). Following the development of chemical tests of bodily substances for alcohol, legislation of the World War II era introduced the tests into the enforcement process by permitting the police to request them and the prosecutors to present the results in court as evidence that the driver had attained the prohibited state of drunkenness or impairment. The earliest of these laws followed the recommendation of the American Medical Association that individuals with BACs of 0.15 percent or more be presumed under the influence and those with BACs under 0.05 percent be presumed not under the influence of alcohol. Drivers with intermediate BACs could be found under the influence if this conclusion was corroborated with other evidence (Voas and Lacey, 1989: 139). The presumptions could be rebutted with contrary evidence concerning the condition of the accused.

More recent laws, termed *per se* laws, have replaced the presumptions with flat prohibitions against driving with BACs exceeding a stipulated level. The switch is analogous to replacing laws against "unreasonable" speeding with set speed limits. Almost all states have now enacted per se laws in addition to classical drunk driving prohibitions. The most common limit is 0.10 percent BAC, but increasing numbers of states are moving to 0.08 percent.

The place of criminal justice in controlling drunk driving

As Williams noted in the statement that begins this chapter, drunk driving policy in America uses law, especially criminal law, as its cornerstone. In order to appreciate the ways in which law exerts its influence, and in order to understand the limits of law in influencing behavior, it is necessary to consider the functions of criminal punishment. Among these can be listed retribution, incapacitation, reform, and general deterrence (see Bean, 1981; Packer, 1968).

The most basic function of criminal punishment, because it legitimizes all the others, is retribution, which may be defined as punishing the evildoer because he has done wrong. Retribution aims at restoring the moral balance. It authorizes punishing the criminal because he deserves to be punished. No utilitarian benefits need be alleged. Even if nothing else were accomplished by punishment—if not a single life could be saved—the retributive principle would justify punishing the wrongdoer. In retributive thinking, if the world were confidently predicted to end tomorrow, the sentences imposed on criminals ought still to be carried out today. As Packer states,

> The retributive position . . . holds, very simply, that man is a responsible moral agent to whom rewards are due when he makes right moral choices and to whom punishment is due when he makes wrong ones. According to this view, these imperatives flow from the nature of man and do not require—indeed do not permit— any pragmatic justification. There is a perceived sense of fitness in the sight of wrongdoers being made to suffer for their misdeeds. [1968: 9]

The retributive principle is most fundamental to criminal law because it provides the legitimate basis for sanctioning offenders. If a crime is committed, punishment is merited. It may be hoped that offenders are changed by the experiences prescribed in their sentences and that society consequently is protected from further mischief. Punishment may also benefit society by providing an example that implicitly warns people to refrain from committing prohibited acts or face the consequences. The punishment of a given offender may be designed with the utilitarian purpose of achieving these extrinsic benefits, but its application must be justified by the blameworthiness of the original deed rather than by the achievement of other goals.

The principle of retribution also limits the punishment that can be applied to an offender. Punishment must be proportionate to the culpability of the conduct (Packer, 1968: 140). If a person has done nothing wrong, then criminal punishments cannot legitimately be applied to him, even though the results might be most beneficial to the person and to society. Minor crimes merit small punishments, and only major crimes merit great ones.

In considering criminal penalties for drunk drivers, it is important to remember both the facilitating and limiting functions of the retributive principle as well as the independence of these functions from goals and restraints posed by utilitarian considerations. On the one hand, if drunk drivers deserve punishment because they have engaged in blameworthy (immoral or dangerous) behavior, their punishment should proceed regardless of whether or not it saves lives. On the other hand, criminal punishments cannot be applied to people who have not committed crimes—that is, who have not been properly arrested, tried, and convicted of an offense—even though we believe that they are dangerous and that the proposed punishment, if applied, would be beneficial. Society's legal arsenal may contain weapons appropriate to the latter case, but criminal law is not among them.

A second set of functions of the criminal law aims to change the offender so that he does not repeat (recidivate) the crime. I call this set reform and include within it the functions traditionally labeled rehabilitation and special deterrence. Rehabilitation uses criminal penalties to transform the offender's motives, creating a lawful citizen out of a law violator. Education and therapy offer possible means to this goal. Education can provide information to those whose criminal acts stem from a lack of knowledge, whereas therapy attempts to resolve psychological conflicts and irrationalities underlying criminal behavior. Although education and therapy are widely provided commodities, among adults they are normally used by those who voluntarily seek them. However, education and therapy can be mandated as part of the drunk driver's punishment through the stipulation of specific programs as conditions of probation. Since the mandate is embodied in a criminal sentence, it assumes a criminal conviction and is justified by the retributive principle, even though the individual is intended to benefit from the programs.

Special deterrence relies on the punishment experience to sensitize the offender to the threat of further punishment for committing a similar crime in the future. In practice, it is difficult to distinguish special deterrent effects from rehabilitative ones, since both are measured by diminished recidivism, but theoretically they are quite different functions. Special deterrence depends on experiences defined as punitive, while rehabilitation depends on experiences defined as beneficial. The distinction is recognized in Packer's equation of special deterrence with intimidation (1968: 45).

Incapacitation differs from rehabilitation and special deterrence in that no attempt is made to change the offender's personality. The offender is placed in a situation in which it is difficult or impossible to act on criminal motives. Incarceration and, in the extreme, capital punishment exemplify sentences that clearly succeed in incapacitating violators of the criminal law. In the field of drunk driving, license actions—suspensions and revocations— may serve to incapacitate offenders without the need for incarceration.

A principal difficulty with reform and incapacitation as mechanisms for dealing with drunk driving (or any other crime) is that they can be

successful only with known offenders, that is, those actually apprehended. In the case of drunk driving, as in that of most crimes, these
individuals form a very small proportion of the target population, so
that even were extremely effective reform and incapacitation techniques available and applied they would not be capable of greatly
reducing the numbers of drunk drivers on the highways. Unfortunately,
this is also true of the population of impaired drivers in fatal crashes.
Only one in six highly intoxicated drivers involved in fatal crashes has
had prior drunk driving convictions and could therefore have been
affected by criminal justice–based programs for reforming or incapacitating offenders (National Highway Traffic Safety Administration,
1991).

The target population of all potential drunk drivers can in theory be
affected by criminal punishment through the function of general deterrence. This refers to the broad threat of the criminal law to punish
those who violate its standards. The threat is reinforced by punishing
convicted offenders, but its effect is expected to be achieved mainly
through its impact on those who are not punished.

General deterrence is a theoretical principle that predicts suppression
of behavior when subjected to a threat perceived as swift, certain, and
severe. The principle is a psychological one, centering on perception.
The perception of a threat may be affected by policies which influence
the objective swiftness, certainty, and severity of punishment. Increases in maximum and average sentences, increments in law enforcement, and streamlining of case processing in courts exemplify changes
in severity, certainty, and swiftness, respectively. At least in the long
run, changes like these should be reflected in changed public perceptions of the legal threat. In addition, perceptions can be affected by
communications. The need for such communications, exemplified by
publicity in mass media, is especially important where real-world
changes are obscure and unlikely to be witnessed in person by most
members of the target population. Increases in severity of punishment
for drunk driving, for example, would be witnessed at firsthand by
only the small fraction of drivers who are apprehended, convicted, and
sentenced for this offense—generally on the order of 1 percent of the
driving population during any year. To affect the perception of all
drivers it would be necessary to publicize the increased punishments
being meted out for drunk driving. In contrast, large increases in certainty of punishment, as might be achieved by a program of investi-

gatory stops of drivers, would be less likely to require publicity, since they would be more evident to the target population in the course of daily activities.

Retributory punishment of drunk drivers

When asked, Americans say that drunk driving is an immoral act meriting criminal punishment. Despite the clear increase in severity of punishments for drunk driving embodied in the legislation of the past decade, numerous polls have found that the public endorses even more severe punishments (see, for instance, General Motors/ *Prevention* Magazine, 1990; McCullough et al., 1990). The sin of the drunk driver is endangering people for reasons not acceptable as excuse or justification, such as to relax, to have fun, or to fit in with the crowd.

Thus there exists a basis for punishing drunk drivers that does not require a showing of deterrent or other effects in order to justify it. However, as previously noted, this basis implies limits on the amount of punishment that can be inflicted. The general answer to the question of how much punishment is merited comes down to how culpable was the criminal act. The question as it relates to drunk drivers is especially difficult to answer because both the culpability and dangerousness of the act of drunk driving can be argued.

The dangerousness of drunk driving

The dominant perception, or typification, of drunk drivers does not fit the majority of drivers impaired by alcohol, including those in serious crashes. The typification implies a high probability of serious injury resulting from every event of drunk driving. However, comparison of the number of alcohol-related fatalities with the estimated number of miles driven by drivers with BACs over 0.10 percent shows that there is less than one fatality for every six hundred thousand impaired miles driven (Voas, 1988a). In comparison with some other activities, including legal ones like motorcycle riding, this may not seem especially dangerous. Most contemporary statutes deliberately overlook evidence that the driving in the specific case may have been safe: "A driver who was operating his vehicle flawlessly and who could pass a field sobriety test would still be guilty of drunk driving if a breath test showed his BAC to be 0.10 or greater" (Jacobs, 1989: 77). If a person has committed an act which is potentially damaging but highly unlikely to have that effect in the specific case, it may be hard to speak of the act as objectively dangerous.

The conclusion that drunk driving is a serious problem can be most directly reached by focusing not on the individual impaired trip, but on the total product of billions of trips with elevated risks of serious crashes. The thousands of lives lost annually in alcohol-related crashes can be deemed not only a national crisis, but a national disgrace. However, the indignation engendered by the adoption of this viewpoint is most legitimately directed at the problem rather than at the individual driver, who must be judged in terms of his own risk rather than the totality of the risk engendered by millions of people. The latter is not a legitimate consideration in determining how much punishment is warranted in the individual case.

Some light can be shed on the dangerousness of drunk driving by considering the comparable behavior of speeding. Breaking the speed limit is the most common violation of the vehicle code. Research has found that where conditions are favorable, such as on well-designed rural highways, the vast majority of drivers engage in this violation (Transportation Research Board, 1984). Moreover, because higher speeds reduce the time available to react to emergencies and increase the amount of damage suffered in crashes, it seems reasonable to regard speeding as a dangerous law violation, other things being equal (Wagenaar, Streff, and Schultz, 1990). Such a conclusion will be evident to someone contemplating the consequences of a high-speed collision and would seem to justify penalizing a surviving driver very heavily. However, the proportion of occasions on which speeding results in crashes is minuscule, and this is reflected in the fact that fines and other consequences meted out to speeders who have not had crashes are trivial. In the absence of strong political forces with an interest in speeding behavior, as contrasted with drunk driving, the issue of speed's harmfulness has been less discussed (but see, for example, Transportation Research Board, 1984, and Wagenaar, Streff and Schultz, 1990). However, the problem of evaluating specific behavior that has a high relative but low absolute risk of a very costly outcome is comparable to that which confounds the student of drunk driving.

The culpability of the drunk driver

It is possible to question the subjective culpability, or blameworthiness, of the drunk driver. Deaths and injuries associated with drunk driving are virtually never intended. If *accidental* is not an appropriate word, *unintended* is. Faced with this issue, courts and legislatures have had little problem in removing the traditional requirement of criminal intent from the drunk driving offense, rendering it a crime of strict liability. Such divergence from traditional criminal procedure is common in traffic law generally; a speeder, for instance, can be found guilty of the offense even though he proves that he honestly and reasonably was complying with the reading on a speedometer that happened to be defective. However, as Jacobs notes, it is extremely unusual for a serious crime bearing heavy penalties to be defined and enforced without regard to evidence of subjective culpability, including at least the showing of negligence on the part of the offender.

In contrast, rather than focus on statistical averages it is possible to view drunk driving in its extreme form. The image of highly dangerous behavior coupled with antisocial attitudes that are contemptuous of life itself is not without real-world models. Although even in these cases it may be difficult to talk of specific intent to harm, gross negligence is likely to be involved, and a category far more serious than traffic offenses is needed to reflect the offender's culpability and therefore the amount of punishment merited.

I believe that the blameworthiness of behavior—and therefore the amount of criminal punishment justified for it—must be judged in the individual case and not as a general matter. The definition used in this book, which includes all impairment that significantly raises the risk of serious crashes, implies that all drunk driving is in some degree blameworthy and deserving of punishment. However, attention to the relationship between BAC and serious crash risk suggests that the degree of culpability should be viewed as a function of the degree of impairment or, indirectly, of the BAC attained in the individual case (Terhune and Fell, 1982), along with such other factors as the presence of traffic and especially of pedestrians, evidence of risky and dangerous maneuvers, and so on. Some impaired drivers may recognize their impairment and attempt to compensate for it by driving more slowly and carefully, thus presenting less of a risk than those who, equally impaired, drive fast and recklessly. Drunk driving, like speeding, is not accurately thought of as a single kind of behavior of uniform dangerousness and blameworthiness. It covers a wide range of both characteristics, and the principle of retribution thus varies in what it demands and permits in the way of legitimate punishments for individual drunk drivers.

Reform and incapacitation of drunk drivers

Attempts at rehabilitation through education and therapy often characterize the sentencing of drunk drivers in America today. Typically, offenders considered to be first-timers are assigned to schools for drunk drivers, the curriculum for which centers on teaching the relationship between alcohol consumption and crash risk. An air of optimism seems to pervade the courses I have sampled as an onlooker (without making any attempts at scientific sampling). Teachers seem to rely on the assumption that their lessons will be effective and that most students will see the error of their ways and not drive again after drinking. I have not come across a curriculum that assumes a large proportion of failures: students who in being apprehended for drunk driving signal the existence of a habit that has a good chance of being repeated, indeed during the course itself. If recidivism were expected, the course could better focus more on offering advice for safer drinking and driving than on providing reasons for not drinking and driving at all. Examples of topics that might appear in the hypothetical curriculum include techniques for reducing peak blood-alcohol concentration, such as drinking more slowly, consuming more diluted drinks, and consuming food before and during drinking (Burns and Moskowitz, 1980). Students might also be taught to compensate for impairment by means such as reducing speed and fastening seat belts.

The therapeutic programs to which most drunk drivers are sentenced are generally low-cost outpatient programs along the lines of group therapy and Alcoholics Anonymous (Stewart and Ellingstad, 1989). The minimal nature of these programs may be due in part to constraints on the extensiveness of involuntary treatment that can be mandated for people found guilty of what may be formally only a traffic offense. It may reflect the inability of most drunk drivers to pay for deep and extensive therapy and the unwillingness of the authorities to subsidize such treatment. Perhaps it also reveals doubts among professionals about what can be accomplished when noncompliant patients are exposed to extensive therapy.

Unfortunately, on the basis of existing research, skepticism over the reformative capability of drunk driving education and therapy is warranted. Perhaps most informative in the evaluation of offender education and therapy is a series of studies comparing educational and therapeutic programs offered to drunk drivers with the alternative of license suspension or revocation. (Participation in these programs is often solicited by offering the offenders retention of licenses that otherwise would have been suspended or revoked.) This line of research was reviewed for the Surgeon General's Workshop by Nichols and Ross (1989; 1990). Among the programs reviewed were a combination of educational and treatment options in California (Hagen, 1977; Hagen et al., 1978; Sadler and Perrine, 1984; Tashima and Peck, 1986) and in Washington State (Salzberg and Klingberg, 1983) and drug and alcohol education in North Carolina (Popkin et al., 1983; Popkin et al., 1988). These studies generally found that drunk drivers experiencing license actions were less likely to recidivate than those assigned to the programs.

The conclusion has been reinforced in a subsequent report from California, a quasi-experimental comparison of convicted drunk drivers penalized in various ways (Tashima and Marelich, 1989). Of all the sanctions studied, license suspension produced the best results in terms of subsequent crashes for first offenders. Among second offenders, the group receiving alcohol treatment programs had considerably more crashes than the suspension group; however, they had fewer alcohol-related crashes, suggesting a possible treatment effect, though not improved overall safety.

A series of evaluations of various educational and therapeutic programs sponsored by the federal Alcohol Safety Action Programs in the 1970s was earlier reviewed by Nichols and his colleagues (e.g., Nichols, Ellingstad and Reis, 1980), with similar conclusions. They noted that the better-designed evaluations were least likely to conclude that the programs were effective.

Nichols has recently summarized the evaluation literature on education and treatment for drunk driving offenders as follows:

The studies indicate that education and treatment programs can affect the offenders exposed to them; however, these effects are limited to reduced DWI arrests or convictions, usually among first-time offenders who have been exposed to educational programs. Evidence of reduced DWI recidivism among repeat offenders has been reported less frequently. There is some evidence that short-term . . . DWI schools may *increase* recidivism among more severe repeat offenders or problem drinkers. [1990: 48]

The literature gives only a modest basis for assuming that education or therapy has an impact on crashes, which ought to be the bottom line for safety programs; yet the apparent ability of some programs to impact rearrests for some kinds of offenders cautions against premature pessimism (see, for instance, Tashima and Marelich, 1989; McKnight and Voas, 1990). There is also the possibility that more effective programs will be developed. In light of the numerous negative evaluations, however, the best explanation for the persistence of most current programs of education and treatment may be the existence of professional lobbies that are committed to them and the organizational need of courts to dispose of large numbers of drunk driving cases economically.

In contrast to the disappointing findings concerning reform, the comparisons just noted suggest that license suspension and revocation policies are effective in incapacitating known drunk-driving offenders. The incapacitating effect of depriving people of their licenses is far from perfect, of course. In various studies, the majority of sanctioned drivers are found to continue driving, a fact made evident both by confessions to interviewers and by the experience of violations and crashes during the period of the license action. However, suspended and revoked drivers appear to accumulate less mileage than they did prior to the actions, and they apparently drive more safely, that is, in a way that is expected not to attract the attention of patrolling police (Ross and Gonzales, 1988).

Furthermore, the superiority in safety-related matters of drunk drivers deprived of their licenses over those permitted to retain them on condition of participating in educational and therapeutic programs appears to last beyond the formal punishment. The reason for this common finding has not been demonstrated, although one possibility is that those deprived of licenses choose not to become relicensed because of the fees, insurance surcharges, and examinations required for relicensing. They have had the benefit of an education lasting several weeks or months in how to drive without a license and without being caught by police. Their continued driving, illegal and uninsured, may maintain the lower mileage and safer style noted among those driving while under suspension and revocation. For whatever reasons, there does seem to be a social gain in the reduced violations and crashes of drivers subjected to license actions, both during and after their punishment.

These advantages seem to be attained without the imposition of an unacceptable economic burden on most offenders' families. Few offenders make credible claims to have lost their jobs, even in jurisdictions with hard license revocation lasting a minimum of three months (Ross and Gonzales, 1988; Wells-Parker and Cosby, 1987; Johnson, 1986). The hardship appears to fall, predictably, mainly upon workers whose jobs require driving, for example, truckers and deliverymen.

The principal reservation that can be raised about the incapacitating function of license actions concerns the ability of those sanctioned to violate the restrictions with impunity. Various innovations have been proposed to increase conformity with the sanctions. One option is to improve the ability of police to identify drivers who are violating the law. For example, license plates for vehicles registered to a person whose driver's license is revoked can be confiscated and replaced with new, identifying, ones. In one version, used in Ohio, the plates are obvious to the public, perhaps adding ignominy to the consequences of a drunk driving conviction. In Minnesota, the plates appear normal but are identifiable to the police by special letters. In either case, any vehicle operator can without further reason be legally stopped and asked to produce a license. Another innovation, designed to assure compliance with the provisions of limited licenses and of probation, is ignition interlocks. These devices prevent starting of a vehicle without giving proof, through a breath test, of a tolerable BAC. Although such devices can be fooled, initial field tests find that they appear to reduce violations of the restrictions (Morse and Elliott, 1990).

In sum, although educational and therapeutic programs have not generally been found to yield safety benefits when applied to drunk drivers, license actions are demonstrably effective in preventing crashes and saving lives. The principal mechanism seems to be incapacitation, rather than reform. Most license-deprived people continue to drive when they think they can get away with it. This means that attention must be given to techniques for enforcing the restrictions prescribed by the license actions.

License suspension and revocation do reduce drunk driving by apprehended offenders. However, even if they were applied universally to all drunk drivers known to the authorities, the contribution to lifesaving through the incapacitation of offenders would be limited by the small proportion of dangerous drunk drivers who are known and who thus can be punished with license actions. What is more, actual programs are capable of achieving only partial incapacitation for those deprived of their licenses.

Deterrence

There is little evidence that criminal punishment can produce special deterrence of convicted drunk drivers. The literature on the effects of jail sentences (Voas, 1986) contains no support for expectations of special deterrence. Indeed, some of the studies reviewed by Voas found that more punitive sentences were associated with worse subsequent safety records, a finding that may in part reflect imperfectly controlled correlations between punishment and both prior and subsequent records. (The drivers with the worst prior records are more likely to be jailed and also more likely to drive badly in the future.) More recent studies have also failed to find evidence of special deterrence; examples include Tashima and Peck (1986) in California, Coleman and Guthrie (1988) on multiple offenders in Minnesota, Ross and Voas (1989) in Ohio, and Martin, Annan, and Forst (1990) on a judicially developed jailing program for first offenders in Minneapolis. Vingilis et al. (1990) found, in a large Canadian city, a positive correlation between the length of jail terms served by repeat-offender drunk drivers and their subsequent alcohol-related collisions: the longer the jail experience, the worse the following performance. In contrast, length of license suspension was negatively related to both total crashes and alcohol-related ones—the longer the suspension, the better the subsequent performance. However, the study was poorly controlled and, as the authors themselves suggest, the relationship may be due in part or entirely to differences in the populations given sentences of different length. In their study of mandatory jail law in Tennessee, Jones et al. (1988), who had initially reported apparently successful special deterrence, concluded that changes in behavior of drivers sent to jail were minor and that the effect was only temporary. The only recent study claiming reformation from the jailing of drunk drivers (Siegal, 1985) dealt with a program that combined jail with a therapeutic intervention unimaginatively titled the Weekend Intervention Program. The optimistic findings of this isolated (and rather weak) study conflict with the general run of results concerning both jail and therapy and therefore by themselves are not strong evidence.

The principal opportunity for criminal law to be effective in reducing drunk driving is, paradoxically, not by affecting the apprehended law violators, who stand within its power. Rather, it lies in affecting unapprehended individuals who are sensitive to the threat that, should they behave illegally, they will be punished. This larger group contains all people who might be able and willing to break the law and who can perceive the threat of punishment for that action. In punishing the apprehended criminal, the justice system is helping to communicate and render credible its more general threat. If the threat is broadly perceived and serves to restrain the threatened activity, general deterrence has been accomplished.

The direct avoidance response to the threat of punishment should be distinguished from long-range behavioral changes that have been posited due to the continued experience of threat over time (Snortum, 1988). Andenaes (1974) speaks of the long-range accomplishment as "general prevention." Prohibitions accompanied by threats of punishment for their violation may lead to the development of parallel social norms, and behavior initially engaged in to avoid the punishment may become habitual over time, so that the threat could be removed but the new behavior—based on habit and supported by social norms— would remain. The achievement of long-range normative and behavioral changes as a consequence of deterrent threats is a plausible expectation (Grasmick and Bursik, 1990), provided that the threats are initially credible. The best evidence of credible threats would be immediate modification of behavior so as to avoid them, that is, simple deterrence. The lack of an immediate response to a threat would suggest a lack of credibility for it, which is hardly likely to render it capable of performing educational or habit-forming functions. Briefly, then, the achievement of general prevention would seem to require the prior achievement of general deterrence.

The classical statement of general deterrence proposes that behavior will be deterred to the extent that it is threatened with punishment perceived to be severe, swift, and certain. Drunk driving policy based on deterrence attempts to provide such punishment and to publicize it so that it is perceived by the target group, the onlookers, rather than just by those apprehended. In recent years, this policy has focused on jail sentences as a means of assuring severity; on administrative process as a means of assuring swiftness; and on liberal and intensive police patrol as a means of assuring certainty of punishment. My discussion will take up each of these in turn.

Severity of punishment

When people demand tough laws concerning drunk driving in America, they are usually speaking of jail sentences for the offenders. In spite of the costliness of this type of punishment and the lack of sufficient facilities to support a credible program of even minimal incarceration for apprehended drunk drivers, who number more than a million every year, American jurisdictions have almost totally ignored the obvious alternative: high fines. This despite their importance, in the form of day-fines based on a percentage of annual income, in the much-admired Scandinavian systems of dealing with drunk driving. At the end of a decade of great concern over punishing drunk drivers, the fines mandated for this offense in America are probably, in constant dollars, at a historic low (Jacobs, 1989). Even the highly publicized first-offender fines of $250 and $350 associated with New York State's STOP-DWI program appear trivial in comparison with the other financial consequences of a drunk driving apprehension, including legal fees and insurance surcharges, and with fines in other countries. In Norway, for example, people apprehended while driving with a BAC of more than 0.05 percent are punished by a fine of 1½ months' salary before taxes, with a minimum of 10,000 Norwegian crowns, or about $1,500. The magnitude of fines in the United States may be such as to trivialize the drunk driving offense.

Indeed, in Jacobs's words, "Incarceration is our dominant sanction; all other sanctions, with the exception of probation (if sanction it be), are treated indifferently, if not scornfully" (1989: 117). The importance of jail sentences in current drunk driving policy is that they affirm the seriousness of the offense, the grave criminality of what has been done. That these coexist with a fine structure that proclaims the opposite— namely, that the offense is a minor one—is but one of many paradoxes characterizing drunk driving policy in America.

It has proved hard to maintain a consistent jailing policy for drunk drivers, especially for first offenders. Imprisonment has traditionally been available in American law as a punishment for driving while intoxicated, but until recently it was virtually never used in routine cases. The pressure to jail drunk drivers intensified in the 1980s, based on the rising consciousness of the problem and its typification as a serious crime. Both the executive and legislative branches of government, strongly affected by the victims' movement, supported widespread increases in severity of prescribed criminal penalties. However, the more severe penalties had to be applied by a judicial branch that often did not see things in the same way. Beyond the tales of victims, judges experienced the commonplace nature of much drunk driving and its frequent failure to result in actual harm. The judiciary also saw moral distinctions between their drunk driving clientele and more traditional criminal types, and they were reluctant to impose punishments that may have struck them as unwarranted from a retributive viewpoint (Robbins, 1986). In addition, the judges could not have failed to be influenced by the inability of jail facilities in most communities to accommodate large increments in their inmate populations.

The characterization of judges' views noted here was not universal. Some individual judges, perhaps as a result of their political views, social philosophy, or personal experiences, agreed that drunk driving was serious criminality deserving of imprisonment. Judge Edward Emmett O'Farrell of New Philadelphia, Ohio, for example, received national attention for a policy of fifteen-day jail sentences for first offenders (Ross and Voas, 1989), and at one point a majority of the bench of Hennepin County (Minneapolis), Minnesota, agreed to jail first offenders for at least two days (Falkowski, 1984). However, on the whole, judges have been reluctant to impose jail sentences on routine drunk-driving offenders.

This judicial diffidence impressed many legislatures as excessively lenient treatment of dangerous criminals. If the judges chose not to use their discretion to sentence in an appropriate way, then the discretion would be removed. In consequence, minimum jail sentences have been mandated in many of the avalanche of drunk driving laws enacted in the 1980s. At present, in part because of incentives provided by the National Highway Traffic Safety Administration, most states mandate either forty-eight hours' jail or equivalent community service for second-offender drunk drivers, and several require jail even for first-timers.

Although mandatory jail laws may have increased the incidence of confinement for drunk drivers, their implementation has been far from complete. Judicial discretion has proved difficult to control. One can mandate a punishment for the guilty, but it is not possible to mandate a finding of guilty for all those charged, and a not uncommon result of mandatory jail laws has been a rise in dismissals and not-guilty findings (Heinzelman, 1985; Ilich, 1986). A close look at judicial response to such laws in Indiana and New Mexico (Ross and Foley, 1987) found that judges sometimes report imposition of jail sentences to motor vehicles authorities but in fact pronounce other sentences. Moreover, drivers actually sentenced to jail sometimes avoid serving the sentences. Studies of jurisdictions that formally mandated jail for first-offender drunk drivers have found noncompliance in proportions ranging from a significant minority of cases (for instance, Jones et al., 1988, in Tennessee) to near totality (Ross, McCleary, and LaFree, 1990, in Arizona).

In my opinion, the first question to ask and answer in order to justify jailing drunk drivers ought to be whether such treatment is warranted on the basis of the dangerousness and blameworthiness of the specific offense. As I indicated above, it is not easy to answer this question, but a case can be made for the affirmative, one capable of supporting specific and even general jailing actions. When looked at in appropriate ways, drunk driving appears to be a serious crime involving gross negligence on the part of the offender and perpetration of harm to others. Nothing more is needed to justify these policies. However, the bulk of the debate concerning jail has concerned not its justifiability, but its deterrent effectiveness.

The fervor with which deterrence has been claimed suggests that many supporters of the policy of jailing drunk drivers may be uncomfortable with basing their support solely on the culpable nature of the behavior and find it necessary to show that lives are being saved through the deterrence mechanism. However, the accumulated research fails to yield much support for claims of general deterrence as a consequence of jailing routine drunk-driving law violators. Little in the way of reduced drunk driving has been found in most studies of enacted jailing policies, and even were an effect assumed, the heavy individual and social costs associated with these policies would weigh against their use when compared with less expensive options.

Claims for the deterrent effectiveness of jailing drunk drivers have often relied on the impression that the Scandinavians have achieved control over drunk driving through such a policy. In fact, adequate scientific evidence for the existence of either short- range or long-range deterrent effects of the Scandinavian laws is lacking (Ross, 1975), and even were the impression confirmed, social and cultural differences between Scandinavian countries and countries like Canada and the United States would caution against the expectation that the same results would occur in the latter countries.

The increasing popularity of mandatory jailing laws in the United States offers a broad and diverse field on which to look for deterrent impacts, and the findings are in general unfavorable. Perhaps the landmark study is that of Tennessee (Jones et al., 1988) because the researchers found that the policy had been fairly well implemented; most convicted drunk drivers were in fact going to jail. A state statute that became effective July 1, 1982, required a 48-hour jail sentence for first-offender drunk drivers, a minimum of 45 days for second offenders, and 120 days for third offenders. No alternative sentences, such as to community service, were provided. Case studies of Chattanooga and Nashville found that "the great preponderance of persons convicted ... are being given jail sentences as the law intended ... in sharp contrast to the situation before the new law when jail sentences were a rarity" (67). Public opinion surveys found that the mandatory jail penalty was fairly well known, though there was "some skepticism that it was actually being imposed" (31). On the basis of statewide fatal crash measures, however, the authors concluded that "the 1982 legislation has had no apparent effect on alcohol-related crashes" (70).

My colleagues and I came to the same conclusion in an analysis of a mandatory jail law for first offenders in Arizona (Ross, McCleary, and LaFree, 1990). Likewise, a study of the fifteen-day first- offender jailing policy in New Philadelphia, Ohio (Ross and Voas, 1989), found the same situation as Jones in Tennessee: evidence that the theoretical preconditions for deterrence were at least partially attained, in that the driving public knew about the law, but no evidence of an actual behavioral effect. These findings also parallel those of some earlier studies of mandatory jail policies in Chicago (Robertson, Rich, and Ross, 1973), Phoenix (Voas, 1975), and an Australian town (Misner and Ward, 1975). Some of these studies found that the policies were poorly implemented, but it is doubtful that the public knew of this. Moreover, the conclusion parallels the one offered for jurisdictions in which jailing policies were well implemented, such as Tennessee (Jones et al., 1988) and Yakima County, Washington (Grube and Kearney, 1980).

The only apparent exception to the negative findings concerning the general deterrent ability of jail sentences for drunk driving in case studies concerns a 1982 attempt by judges in Hennepin County (Minneapolis), Minnesota, to secure, through mutual agreement, a uniform two-day jail sentence for first-offender drunk drivers. Although a few judges refused to join in the agreement, the policy was fairly well applied. For more than two years, 80 percent of first-time offenders received the agreed-upon jail sentence. Evaluations by Falkowski (1984) and Cleary and Rodgers (1986), both of which used interrupted time-series analysis, found a possible intervention effect in indexes of drunk driving. However, Falkowski's claim of deterrence as a consequence of the judicial policy is greatly weakened by the fact that the changes did not occur at the inception of the local policy, as deterrence theory would predict, but rather following an unexplained lag of two months, to almost precisely the date at which a major package of state laws relating to drunk driving came into effect. The possible causal role of the latter was stressed by Cleary and Rodgers. It appears that something affected drunk driving in Minnesota in 1982, but the Hennepin County jailing policy is only one among many possible causes. Claims of the effectiveness of the jailing policy are favored by the fact that the change was greater in Minneapolis than elsewhere in the state. However, the unexplained time lag and the plausibility of an alternative explanation in the passage of state laws streamlining the administrative process for driver-license penalties vitiate the case for the deterrent explanation. Added to this is the fact that Hennepin County otherwise stands alone in the field of case studies in claiming a deterrent effect for jailing drunk drivers.

A deterrent effect for jail has been claimed in research based on an analysis of statistical data from multiple states. A regression analysis of fatal crashes in the forty-eight contiguous states (Zador et al., 1989) found that first-offender mandatory jail or community service laws were related to lower rates of alcohol-involved fatal crashes. (Other laws with significant negative relationships to these crashes included administrative license actions, which appeared to have a greater effect than jail, and "illegal *per se*" statutes, which appeared to have an effect of the same magnitude as the jail laws.) The modest nature of the benefits was noted as follows:

The current analysis indicates that *per se* laws, administrative license suspension, and first-offense jail/community service sentencing reduced driver involvement in fatal crashes nationally by about 0.8 percent in 1980 and about 1.4 percent in 1982, a change of 0.6 percent. Thus, enactment of the three types of laws studied here can account for only about one quarter of the reduction potentially attributable to alcohol programs in those years. [Zador et al., 1989: 19–20]

Analyses like this attempt to control the other causal factors acting in real-life situations by a combination of statistical adjustment for the estimated effect of specific rival causes and subtraction of the effect of general conditions found in comparison jurisdictions. Which specific control variables are chosen and how they are measured are difficult and debatable matters, as is the choice of comparison jurisdictions. The adequacy of the adjustments made in any study can be criticized, as it was for the Zador et al. study by Klein (1989: 20–22). The weaknesses inherent in any specific study of this type can be compensated for if similar findings appear in replications using somewhat different methods. For the case at issue, replications exist in an analysis of trends in fatality data in states with and without mandatory jail (among other laws) by Joksch (1988), and in a set of interrupted time-series analyses of single-vehicle nighttime fatal crash data, related to different combinations of drunk driving provisions in the various states (Klein, 1989). The Klein study, methodologically the stronger of the two replications, supports the Zador et al. study in its finding of a deterrent effect for administrative license actions but does not find an effect for jail. The Joksch study finds no effect for laws of either type.

In sum, the multistate literature includes one study supporting the claim of a deterrent effect for jail, but two finding no support. All the case study literature on jailing policies, except that on the 1982 Hennepin County judicial agreement, is negative, and both analyses of the latter are best interpreted as providing evidence that something beneficial may have occurred, but not as providing unambiguous testimony for the deterrent effect of mandatory jail laws.

The overall negative findings on the deterrent effects of severe punishment disconfirm not only theory but also intuition. They invite speculation as to why expected results were not found. I believe that the most plausible reason for the inability of jail threats to deter drunk drivers lies in the very small actual and perceived chances of being caught. Nowhere in the United States is there good reason for a driver to think that a given trip taken while illegally impaired by alcohol is likely to result in apprehension, much less prosecution and conviction, for drunk driving. Estimates of the actual chance of apprehension for a drunk driver in America are on the order of one chance or less in one thousand occasions or five thousand impaired miles driven (Summers and Harris, 1978; Voas, 1988a). Although surveys suggest that the risk perceived by the public is considerably (and unrealistically) higher, it may still not be high enough for would-be drunk drivers to take the threat seriously. The inducements to drive drunk in America are, as previously noted, numerous and strong: we are committed to drinking and we are committed to driving. In light of these inducements, the threat posed by the legal system is too remote to demand attention. The chance of punishment can be viewed as virtually nil, and if people believe they will never be caught, why should they care what the punishment might be?

This explanation is compatible with the fact of little scientific evidence for a deterrent effect from mandatory jail laws. It is also compatible with the experience of reductions in indexes of drunk driving simultaneous with the announcement of major increases in enforcement efforts. It is furthermore compatible with the common finding of decay in these achievements over time as the target population experiences the actual, generally very low, levels of risk in their aftermath (Ross, 1982).

Whether or not jailing policies will eventually be found to have deterrent consequences, they constitute a costly approach to handling drunk drivers. The costs include the pain and suffering of the prisoner, a negative from the utilitarian viewpoint although possibly a plus from the viewpoint of retribution. Beyond this, the adoption of policies emphasizing jail—and the consequent raising of the ante for conviction of drunk driving—has resulted in increased workloads for the courts and therefore longer delays in processing of the offenders. Where defendants are nonetheless convicted, limited corrections facilities are often strained (Voas, 1975; Ross, 1976; National Institute of Justice, 1984). These consequences may not be inevitable; Falkowski, for example, found that the Hennepin County program did not overwhelm the jail, where, as noted by Lewis (1990), there was ample space prior to the program's inception. However, in light of the generally negative evidence concerning the deterrent accomplishments of jail, the costliness of the policy reinforces the wisdom of looking to other kinds of sanctions (such as fines and license actions) for handling routine drunk driving offenses, provided that these satisfy the criminal law's retributive goals.

Swiftness of punishment

Criminal justice is not merely costly; it is slow. Some slowness in the process is inherent and necessary to permit the due process of law with which the individual is protected against the superior power of the state in criminal proceedings. From the viewpoint of retribution, it is important that the punished individual shall have been found guilty of culpable conduct in a process that provides him with procedural protections as well as a strong benefit of doubt when the evidence is ambiguous. However, from the viewpoint of deterrence, a slow process is regrettable. The deterrent effectiveness of any punishment is expected to be a function of the swiftness with which it is perceived to be delivered. Delay in the punishing of offenders, however necessary from other viewpoints, threatens to weaken the ability of the criminal justice system to deter.

Increasing the swiftness of punishment, unlike increasing the severity, has not been a central preoccupation in traditional drunk driving policy. One reason may be the lesser ability of swiftness to satisfy the retributive function of criminal justice. Another is the difficulty of devising policies for the purpose of reducing delay in punishing drunk drivers, since use of the criminal justice system entails inherently cumbersome procedures. Thus, few opportunities for evaluating the impact of swift punishment have been available in the realm of drunk driving.

It has only been with the realization that legal opportunities to penalize drunk drivers exist outside of criminal justice that swiftness-related interventions and evaluations have become possible. The key to opportunity lies in the fact that a meaningful source of punishment for drivers lies in depriving them of their licenses, and this can be accomplished by administrative as well as judicial action. If the Department of Motor Vehicles issues the license, then the department can take it away. Considerations of due process are not totally ignored, for the driver's license has been recognized constitutionally as an "important interest" that cannot be denied lightly. However, the constraints applied by administrative due process are less demanding than those of criminal due process, and the criterion for proving the offense is the preponderance of evidence, rather than proof beyond a reasonable doubt. Indeed, the scope and power of the administrative process are enormous: it can sanction and restrain dangerous behavior through the use of analogues to nearly all powers of the criminal court, except that to imprison. Besides that, it has the potential to act quickly and decisively.

Administrative license withdrawal was for many years used as a tool to induce drivers to cooperate with breath test procedures. Drivers *refusing* a police officer's demand for a test might count on defeating a drunk driving criminal charge, but so-called implied consent statutes permitted punishing them with revocation of their driving licenses in consequence. However, if a driver took the test and failed it, his punishment, if any, would follow only on completion of a lengthy and uncertain criminal prosecution. Beginning with Minnesota in 1976, modern "administrative per se" statutes also penalized *failing* the breath test with license withdrawal. Drivers were thus punished quickly and certainly, apart from whatever might happen in the parallel criminal case. Typically, the motivation to cooperate in the procedure was maintained by making the period of disqualification for refusal longer than that for cooperating and failing in the test.

The realization that the administrative process might be useful in deterring drunk drivers has come comparatively recently, and not all jurisdictions have administrative per se laws yet. In some states, opposition by criminal-defense lawyers, along with misgivings and perhaps even jealousies on the part of the judiciary in the matter of sharing sanctioning power with administrators, have stalled adoption of such laws. However, the commonsensical and theoretical advantages of increasing the swiftness of punishment for drunk drivers have led most states to adopt a variation of administrative per se. Several evaluations now available generally support the ability of these laws to save lives.

There are numerous differences from state to state in the provisions of administrative license suspension or revocation laws. The presence of such discrepancies suggests that both the certainty and the swiftness of punishment actually delivered differ among the states, and that the impact of these laws on drunk driving varies accordingly. In general, the laws provide that licenses may be seized by the police if a driver properly accused of drunk driving either refuses an evidentiary breath test or completes it and shows an illegal BAC. All the laws allow a limited period of continued driving privileges following seizure of the license, during which an administrative hearing may be demanded and must be granted. An unfavorable administrative review can in all cases be appealed to a court. However, the laws differ on such important matters as the length of the time during which driving privileges are retained and whether they are retained pending an appeal of an administrative finding supporting the police. In some states the driving privileges are completely lost for the duration of the sanction (generally ninety days on a first offense); in others a suspended driver may be granted limited privileges such as driving to and from work; in still others periods of both hard and soft suspension are included. The laws differ over the consequences of technical errors in procedure, such as a failure of the police officer to sign the ticket at the scene, and in whether the arresting or testing officers must appear in person at the administrative hearing. In some states, administrative license revocation procedures work smoothly, whereas in others the machinery is close to being overwhelmed by the case load (Ross, 1991).

Whatever the formal and operational differences among statutes, administrative license actions frequently have been shown to be successful in reducing drunk driving. As noted previously, several studies have concluded that license actions reduce recidivism through incapacitation of the offenders, although this incapacitation is incomplete (e.g., Hagen, 1977; Blomberg, Preusser, and Ulmer, 1987; Sadler and Perrine, 1984). Crashes and violations are much less frequent following license actions than following such alternatives as educational and therapeutic programs. More important, laws providing for administrative license revocation have in many cases been associated with overall reductions in crashes indexing drunk driving, suggesting that general deterrence may be achieved. Formal evaluations have been done in Minnesota, the first state to implement administrative license actions as a keystone in drunk driving policy, where the study focused on a tightening of the law in 1982 (Cleary and Rodgers, 1986); in Wisconsin, where both administrative and judicial revocation processes were applicable (Blomberg, Preusser, and Ulmer, 1987); in North Carolina, where the length of suspension was a mere ten days (Lacey, Stewart, and Rodgman, 1984); in Alabama, where license revocation was first mandated, then made discretionary, and then mandatory once more

(Maghsoodloo, Brown, and Greathouse, 1985); and in New Mexico, where deterrent results appeared to have been achieved despite negligible efforts to publicize the deterrent threat (Ross, 1987a). In a complex study with some design problems, administrative revocation laws in Louisiana and North Dakota were judged to have had deterrent effects, though one in Mississippi failed to show results (Stewart, Gruenewald, and Roth, 1989). Beyond these formal evaluations, reductions in alcohol-related or nighttime fatal crashes have been reported as being simultaneous with the adoption of administrative license suspension or revocation laws in Colorado, Illinois, Indiana, Minnesota, Nevada, North Carolina, North Dakota, Oregon, West Virginia, and other states (Nichols and Ross, 1990: 51).

Administrative license revocation laws have also been found to be effective by two (Zador et al., 1989, and Klein, 1989) of the three multistate statistical analyses referred to above. These were the best designed of the three. In both, administrative license revocation laws were found to be the most effective of those categories of laws judged to have any effect. On the basis of Klein's analysis, the National Highway Traffic Safety Administration (1991) has estimated that 364 additional lives would have been saved in 1989 if the twenty-one states lacking administrative license revocation laws had adopted them prior to that year.

Administrative revocation laws have also been found to be cost-effective. For instance, annual savings due to fewer fatalities in nighttime crashes as a consequence of these laws have been estimated at more than $37 million in Nevada, $89 million in Illinois, and more than $100 million in Mississippi. These savings clearly overwhelm the administrative expenses of $201,000, $852,000, and $56,000, respectively. Moreover, the administrative costs are offset in part by offender-paid fees and federal grants (Lacey, Jones, and Stewart, 1991).

In conclusion, it seems clear that administrative license revocation laws not only succeed in incapacitating the offenders to whom they are applied, but also reduce serious crashes and alcohol-related crashes among the general driving population. The theoretical explanation for this phenomenon is general deterrence due to the increased swiftness of punishment following the offense as well as possibly increased certainty of punishment associated with the lower administrative standard of proof compared with the criminal one. Although more research is needed, especially to determine which variations of administrative license action are the most effective and least costly, these laws can be recommended for jurisdictions that currently lack them, with the expectation that they will save lives.

Certainty of punishment

Punishment for the drunk driver in America does not lack in severity. In the words of Voas and Lacey (1989: 137), "[F]rom the early years of this century, the United States has treated [drunk driving] as seriously as any nation in the world." This is true, despite the persistence of fairy tales in the press that associate obscene punishments with drunk driving in places like Bulgaria, South Africa, and even Britain ("Folklore in Traffic Safety," 1989). Although the BACs tolerated in most states are relatively liberal by world standards, some American practices such as mandatorily jailing first offenders would seem incredibly severe to people in most countries. To the extent that the sentences are served in typical American county jails, they may be considered more severe even than the much longer sentences often prescribed in Norway or Sweden, where conditions in correctional institutions accepting drunk drivers more closely resemble those of a budget motel in this country. License actions are also very likely experienced as far more painful in America than in most other countries owing to the more limited range of alternatives to automobile transportation in most of the United States.

With the advent of administrative license revocation laws, the punishment for drunk drivers in America probably comes as swiftly as anywhere in the world. In most countries, drunk drivers are processed exclusively in a criminal justice system, with inevitable procedural delays. Formal sanctions await the resolution of the criminal case. In contrast, administrative sanctions can be regarded as being applied either at the time the license is taken at the scene of the arrest or a few days later when driving privileges are in fact lost. In either case, the delay in the application of the administrative penalty is generally much shorter than that associated with criminal punishments.

From the perspective of deterrence, then, objective swiftness and severity of threatened punishment for drunk drivers are relatively well achieved in many American states. A driver who is apprehended by a policeman and either refuses or fails an alcohol breath test can count on swift and severe punishment.

The Achilles' heel of deterrent policies aimed at drunk driving, in

America and many other countries, is the law violator's low probability of apprehension and therefore of experiencing any punishment at all. In an elaboration of deterrence theory, Tittle and Rowe (1974), after studying data on crime rates and the certainty of arrest, hypothesized that certainty of punishment must reach a critical threshold level before a deterrent threat can be effective in reducing the crime rate. The need to exceed such thresholds is plausible for all three deterrence variables, but with sanctions like mandatory jail and processes like administrative license revocation one may assume that thresholds for severity and swiftness of punishment are safely exceeded in the typical American jurisdiction, leaving certainty alone at issue.

The probability of arrest for drunk driving in America has been variously calculated. The classic general estimation, by Summers and Harris (1978), is that the objective risk of apprehension for a driver with a BAC exceeding 0.10 percent is about 1 in 2,000. Given that a doubling of drunk driving arrests has occurred nationally since the mid-1970s, a current estimation with these procedures would point to a 1/1,000 risk. Higher risk estimates have been obtained in jurisdictions that make special efforts in drunk driving law enforcement. For example, during the Kansas City Alcohol Safety Action Project in the early 1970s, Beitel, Sharp, and Glauz (1975) calculated the probability of arrest for a driver with a BAC over 0.10 percent as about 1 in 200, and a similar objective risk was calculated by Hause, Voas, and Chavez (1980) during the Stockton, California, Increased D.U.I. Enforcement Project later in the decade. These represent the highest scientifically validated levels of objective risk of apprehension for drunk drivers in the literature.

Since perceived rather than actual risk is the theoretically relevant deterrence variable, driver surveys are the most appropriate means for understanding the level of certainty of punishment. The general finding is that drivers see a risk of apprehension that is higher than the objective one, but still rather low in absolute terms. For example, a telephone survey of Indiana drivers found more than two-thirds estimating the drunk driver's chance of punishment to be less than 1 in 10 (Vargus, 1985), and about 6 in 10 patrons leaving college bars in State College, Pennsylvania (well over half with illegal BACs), considered their chances to be 10 percent or less (Brightly, 1985). Much lower perceived risk levels were found in a Canadian government study (Bragg and Cousins, 1979), where volunteer subjects estimated the probability of being stopped on an impaired trip at about 1/1500, and the probability of being arrested if stopped at about 1/200. The perceived probability of arrest for drunk driving in that study was stated to rank somewhere between the probability of snow in June and that of winning the Olympic Lottery.

These observations lead to the hypothesis that increased deterrence may be best achieved by raising the objective and, presumably in consequence, the perceived risk of punishment. The most direct route to this goal is to increase the quantity and quality of law enforcement. The coincidence of rising arrest rates with falling rates of drunk driving since the mid-1970s, documented in chapter 2, is consistent with this hypothesis, although the evidence is inconclusive, given the numerous other developments associated with a decade of concern for drunk driving. More can be learned from evaluations of recent programs that have increased resources devoted to enforcing drunk driving law.

Perhaps the most important information concerning the deterrent potential of increased law enforcement comes not from American examples, but from the adoption of Random Breath Testing in the Australian states of New South Wales and Tasmania. This experience has been extensively reviewed by Homel in his book, *Policing and Punishing the Drinking Driver* (1988), and in a more recent chapter-length updating (Homel, 1989). The Australian experience is enlightening because of its scope and duration.

The intervention initially consisted of permitting police to set up unannounced checkpoints for the purpose of enforcing the drunk driving law. The procedure is better described as arbitrary than as random:

> Motorists passing a check-point, which are [*sic*] designed to be highly visible, are pulled over for a preliminary roadside breath test in a more or less haphazard manner, and all drivers pulled over are asked to take a test, regardless of the type of vehicle or their manner of driving. . . . Drivers who are positive on the screening test are detained for an evidential breath test." [Homel, 1989: 4]

No judgment is made by the police as to the likelihood that the driver has been drinking. The test is given to all drivers stopped at the checkpoint.

Tests are given in enormous numbers, too. In New South Wales, where the evaluations have been most complete, two hundred extra police were recruited for highway patrol work at the inception of the

Random Breath Testing Program in 1982. The police have administered approximately one million breath tests annually in a driving population of three million, a ⅓ fraction in twelve months. After the first year the traffic police were instructed that each patrol vehicle should carry out one hour of random breath testing per shift.

Extensive publicity was given to the program from its inception. The publicity included paid, professional advertisements as well as unpaid news coverage. Direct experience as well as mass communications also helped to bring perceived levels of increased risk into accord with the fact. By 1987, more than half of Sydney motorists had experienced at least one test, and more than four out of five reported having seen the program in action.

There was a sharp decline in fatal crashes in New South Wales coincidental with the inception of Random Breath Testing. Lives saved amounted to approximately 20 percent, overall. Unlike most previously reported cases, including the classic Cheshire (England) Breathalyser Blitz (Ross, 1977), the numbers of fatal crashes have remained lower over time, with only a minor increase toward prior levels after five years (Homel, 1988: 119). It may be premature to call the accomplishment permanent, but its duration has been extraordinary.

Homel's evaluation attempted to show that police activity in New South Wales led to the experience of testing on the part of large proportions of drivers; that this experience led to perception of a greater risk of arrest and punishment; that this perception led to behavioral change, including changes in drinking and driving habits; and that changes in these habits led to fewer drunk driving occasions and therefore to fewer casualties. On the whole, the evidence supports these linkages and thus the utility of deterrence theory for understanding and guiding policy in the circumstances of the Australian intervention.

The New South Wales experience suggests that increasing the certainty of punishment for drunk drivers was able to produce general deterrent effects. This was the case even though the penalties consisted mainly of fines and license actions and seldom if ever encompassed jail sentences. Homel adds the caution, which he underlines in the original, that "full random testing is also not capable of achieving long-term reductions in casualties unless it is rigorously enforced and extensively advertised" (1989: 30). This is because deterrence appears to be "an unstable process at the individual level, with peer pressure, lack of exposure to RBT, and successful drink-driving episodes operating to erode perceptions and behavior patterns built up through earlier exposure to RBT" (1989: 32).

The Australian experience is not directly applicable to what might be achieved in America, in part because the procedure in detail would violate constitutional guidelines in federal and many state jurisdictions (National Highway Traffic Safety Administration, 1983; Voas and Lacey, 1989). Moreover, the fact of different social environments cautions against unqualified expectations of effectiveness for the techniques, even were they constitutionally acceptable. Related, but less discretionary approaches have been tried in the United States in the last several years, and the general concept of stopping all drivers at road blocks or sobriety checkpoints to observe their behavior as a basis of drunk driving enforcement was approved by the U.S. Supreme Court in *Michigan Dept. of State Police v. Sitz* (1990).

In the context of the New South Wales program, American checkpoint programs appear restrained, even timid. However, they do provide some encouragement for the utility of checkpoints or comparable increments in law enforcement to secure deterrent results. Arizona introduced drunk driving checkpoints as early as 1983 and provided an evaluation for them (Epperlein, 1985). Two checkpoints were mounted on December weekends in each of three patrol areas. There was a sharp and significant decrease in fatal and injury-producing crashes, but not in property-damage crashes, which are less likely to involve alcohol as a factor. However, the checkpoints and their impacts were both temporary and left no lasting consequences.

Checkpoints were also involved in enforcement and information programs in Clearwater and Largo, Florida, and in Indianapolis in the mid-1980s (Lacey et al., 1990). Again, their introduction appears to have been restrained—there were twelve checkpoints in the Florida area and six in Indianapolis. In both areas, surveys confirmed increased awareness of enforcement, and in Florida the survey respondents reported behavioral changes. In Florida, there was a 20 percent decline in alcohol-related crashes and an 8 percent decline in nighttime crashes. The latter criterion is preferable because it averts the need to accept police decisions concerning the involvement of alcohol, an important consideration when the police know that an experiment to reduce alcohol involvement is in progress. Indianapolis also experienced a significant decline in nighttime crashes. It must be remembered that these evaluations are of complex programs involving a great many innovations other than checkpoints.

The most intensive experience with checkpoints in the United States occurred in Charlottesville, Virginia, during 1984 (Voas, Rhodenizer, and Lynn, 1985). In one year, police set up ninety-four checkpoints and stopped twenty-four thousand drivers, an intensity comparable to that in New South Wales. Surveys showed a broad awareness of the checkpoints, and there was an initial increase in the perceived risk of arrest, though it did not change during the course of the year; the median estimate of being caught when over the BAC limit but not "in trouble" driving was 1/100, and when both over the limit and in trouble it was 1/10.

An effect of the Charlottesville checkpoint program on crashes is suggested, but the evidence is ambiguous. There were six criterion variables, all involving "alcohol-related" accidents and thus police judgments. All showed changes in the predicted direction. In the words of the evaluators, the data were "consistent with the hypothesis that the checkpoint program reduced crashes related to drunken driving approximately 10 percent. However, the limited data . . . do not permit a final conclusion, because . . . only three of the six were statistically significant" (46). They expressed disappointment in the small size of the apparent reduction in alcohol-related crashes, contrasted with large changes in public knowledge and attitudes.

An important feature of well-implemented checkpoints is their general visibility and thus their potential to influence the perception of enforcement. In a telephone survey in Charlottesville, half of all drivers "at risk" (who drink) stated that they had seen the checkpoints, and nearly nine in ten knew of the special program. This parallels findings in a study of two Washington-area jurisdictions, one of which had checkpoints, the other historically a higher drunk-driver arrest rate. Residents of both areas thought the former had the higher risk of arrest (Williams and Lund, 1984).

Techniques of enhanced enforcement other than checkpoints have also been found promising for deterring drunk driving. For instance, special drunk driving enforcement personnel were provided for several periods over 3½ years in Stockton, California (Voas and Hause, 1983). The patrols produced sevenfold and tenfold increases in drunk driving arrests during the hours of their operation. While daytime crashes, relatively unlikely to involve alcohol, increased 13 percent during the project period, weekend night crashes, more likely to involve alcohol, declined by 15 percent, and weekday night crashes declined by 10 percent. The introduction of data from comparison cities strengthened confidence in the findings, as did the results of voluntary breath tests of drivers on the roads. Telephone surveys showed broad public awareness of the project. Interestingly, although the extra patrols were limited to specific areas, the changes noted were citywide.

In sum, there is considerable evidence that increasing the actual certainty of punishment for drunk drivers in ways that also ensure adequate publicity can effect reductions in drunk driving. The best evidence at this time comes from the Australian interventions, which cannot be precisely duplicated in the United States because of constitutional problems. In addition, U.S. police forces have been reluctant to mount extensive checkpoint campaigns despite the Supreme Court's approval of the necessary stops. One possible reason is that the yield of offenders in proportion to people questioned is much smaller with checkpoints than with traditional patrol, which is based on such suspicious behavior as weaving across the center line of a road. Police culture traditionally values catching criminals, an accomplishment easily demonstrated in arrest statistics, whereas successful deterrence is hard to demonstrate and may be regarded by many police as mere theory.

Constitutionally acceptable checkpoint programs have been mounted in several American jurisdictions, and available evaluations offer hope for their effectiveness if police can be convinced that they are worth doing. The same optimism can be expressed about other approaches to increasing the actual risk of apprehension for drunk drivers, when accompanied by adequate publicity (see Mercer, 1985). These observations accord with the theoretical expectation that deterrence is a function of the perceived certainty of punishment, and that effective deterrence can be achieved only when this perception exceeds a threshold level.

The limits of deterrence

The bulk of relevant social science literature suggests that deterrence-based law can be of use in saving lives now lost because of drunk driving. Reasonable and credible threats belong in the arsenal of drunk driving countermeasures, on the grounds that they can independently reduce drunk driving and that they may interact with and reinforce countermeasures arising from other perspectives. For example, if subsidized taxis are provided to induce people not to drive on drinking occasions, their use may be enhanced by the presence of a credible threat of punishment if the opportunity goes unused and a drunk driving incident occurs instead.

However, wise policy choices require acknowledgment of the limits of deterrence. A principal one is that infliction of punishment is painful and costly. Even the sinner's suffering is, according to utilitarian reasoning, a negative, which can be tolerated only because of compensating gains. Besides, the costs of rendering deterrent threats credible through adequate enforcement may be beyond the ability or willingness to pay of many U.S. jurisdictions. Low probabilities of apprehension, slow processing, and lenient treatment of offenders owing to limited resources may defeat gains initially achieved by deterrence-based laws.

Beyond this, it appears that many drunk drivers are members of social categories that theory predicts are especially difficult to deter (Zimring and Hawkins, 1973). The conditions of lower-class life in industrial societies seem to lead to preferences for risk over safety and for immediate as against deferred gratification. Such attitudes may diminish the subjective severity and neutralize the perceived swiftness and certainty of punishment. The fact that the Scandinavian countries, which have low rates of drunk driving, experience large fractions of traffic deaths and injuries associated with alcohol suggests that those who remain undeterred are especially likely to experience serious crashes (Ross, 1975: 297).

Perhaps the major limit of the deterrent approach to drunk driving lies in its failure to address the causes of the problem in the socially derived motivation underlying the behavior in question. We attempt to deter behavior by severing the link between motivation and action. The motivation to engage in dangerous behavior is countered by a threat of punishment, but there is no direct attempt to reduce the motivation. Successful deterrence can be accomplished without knowing or understanding why people wish to engage in the prohibited behavior, but alternative approaches attempt to reduce the motivation through manipulating its social sources. Success in this endeavor requires a correct understanding of the institutional causes of the problematic behavior. Options based on this approach will be discussed in subsequent chapters.

The criminal justice system helps maintain the perception that the moral balance of the world is in order, that bad people receive their due. In validating the expectation that evil should not go unpunished, punishment can help people feel better when they experience the effects of evil. It can help them cope with grief and ensure loyalty to a society which, like all others, incurs hurt and tragedy in the course of normal operations. This is the criminal law's retributive function. Beyond this, law and criminal justice have the potential to reduce drunk driving and thus to save lives.

If today we are pessimistic about the reformative ability of the criminal justice system, we can be relatively optimistic concerning its incapacitative function. In the matter of drunk driving, a relatively simple and cheaply applied sanction—license suspension or revocation—is capable of producing important reductions in the rates of further law violation and crash involvement. This despite the rather unpromising clientele—by definition convicted of drunk driving and often having poor records of prior driving performance. If the incapacitating effect is not perfect, it is important. Unlicensed individuals may continue to drive, but they reduce their mileage and drive more prudently.

Reform and incapacitation, however, even if perfectly achieved, could not affect the vast bulk of drunk driving, for they can be applied only to individuals who have come to the attention of the authorities. Most drunk drivers, including five out of six of those destined to kill in alcohol-related crashes, are not known to the authorities, and their behavior cannot be affected by techniques limited to convicted offenders. We must look to the broader effects of the law in order to maximize its usefulness in controlling the dangerous behavior which is the subject of this book.

The principal contribution of criminal justice to saving lives now lost to drunk driving must come through general deterrence, that is, through provision of a credible threat that will cause individuals to refrain from drinking and driving despite the inducements to the behavior that are built into their social environment. This effect can be experienced by drivers who have had no personal contact whatsoever with law enforcement, since their understanding of the consequences of the prohibited act can be affected by information that increases the credibility of the criminal threat.

In contradiction to the principal strain of contemporary policy in this area, there appears to be little if any benefit from increasing the severity of drunk driving penalties beyond what they are today in the United States. Increasing the swiftness of the threatened punishment can be effective, as seen in numerous studies of the adoption of administrative process centering on license actions. Paradoxically, it may be advisable to *reduce* the severity of punishment for at least some drunk drivers by eschewing jail sentences, so their punishment can be handled administratively. This would maximize the swiftness and certainty of penalties in routine cases and free the criminal-justice system from the burden of routine so it can concentrate resources on more extreme and problematic cases.

There is opportunity for the criminal threat to be more effective through an increase in enforcement. Whether this be safety checkpoints or increments in traditional patrol, it appears to promise a significant increment in the benefits available through the law and criminal justice.

Although criminal and other legal punishments can reduce drunk driving and save lives, the system that supports legal threats is costly and inherently limited in effectiveness. It produces social "bads" that have to be borne rather than "goods" to be used and enjoyed and does not act on the causes of drunk driving. Effective deterrent programs may also require resources at the limit of political acceptability. It is insufficient merely to up the ante for being caught, if the chances of apprehension are negligible. Even well-conceived and well-implemented legal threats may leave some populations relatively unaffected, and these resistant populations are likely to be the most dangerous ones. Deterrence thus cannot be the whole of drunk driving policy. It should be conceived as one element in an arsenal of countermeasures, along with other measures based on valid understandings of the social causes of the problem.

Countermeasures Based in Alcohol Policy

Countermeasures based in alcohol policy assume that drunk driving can be reduced by reducing the amount of alcohol consumed in society. If virtually all transportation is accomplished through the use of private automobiles, a decline in overall alcohol consumption and thus in BACs of drivers will reduce crash risks and save lives.

This result is not logically necessary; if all drinking occasions were separated from those of driving or if driving were done only by abstainers, one would not expect reduced crashes regardless of changes in total alcohol consumption. However, the assumption seems to be empirically true in the United States. The private automobile is the chief means of transportation to and from drinking locations outside of the home, and the custom of drivers refraining from drinking in order to provide safe transportation for themselves and their friends is not general in the society. Our highways are lined with drinking establishments that cannot easily be reached other than by car; impairing amounts of alcoholic beverages are routinely consumed there by the patrons. Indeed, the automobile in its capacity as a site of leisure activities itself often serves as a drinking location, and this function is potentially facilitated by such institutions as drive-up liquor stores and gasoline service stations offering cold beer for sale. Drunk driving, in the sense of driving while significantly impaired by alcohol, is a predictable consequence of this life-style. It is equally predictable that, if the life-style is modified to reduce the extent of drinking, the amount of drunk driving may be reduced.

Countermeasures based in alcohol policy that

4

are undertaken to reduce drunk driving will produce additional benefits to the extent that they impact other social problems associated with alcohol consumption. These include several important causes of death in addition to drunk driving. According to the Centers for Disease Control (1990), nearly one hundred thousand people died of alcohol-related causes in 1987, only about a fifth of these in highway crashes. Almost eighteen thousand people died in suicides and homicides in which alcohol was involved, and about fifty thousand died from liver cirrhosis and other intestinal diseases, cancers, cardiovascular diseases, and respiratory diseases, all related to alcohol. Large proportions of deaths caused by drownings, falls, and fires are associated with alcohol. Moreover, alcohol is related to a variety of crimes against the person (Collins, 1981), including assaults on spouses, children, friends, and strangers. Wherever violence is found in America, alcohol is a common accompaniment and presumable causal factor. Like drunk driving, these problems may diminish as a consequence of reduced alcohol consumption.

The realization that drunk driving is part of a larger problem related to the presence of alcohol in society provides an additional justification for using alcohol policy as a source of countermeasures. The benefits are greater insofar as other manifestations of the larger problem are coincidentally reduced, and the costs allocated to drunk driving can be regarded as less by their apportionment among multiple achievements. It also stands to reason that drinking-reduction policies stimulated by an interest in other social problems may beneficially impact drunk driving.

Acknowledgment of a gamut of alcohol-related problems is not inconsistent with acknowledgment that alcohol is valued in American society and that the public perceives benefits from its use. Among the benefits are "increased sociability, interpersonal skills, social assertion, feelings of power, arousal, and tension reduction" (Snortum, Kremer, and Berger, 1987: 243). Discouraging alcohol consumption reduces these benefits, even though it can be argued that overall welfare is increased. Drinking reductions are thus resisted politically, not only by manufacturing and trade interests, but by large segments of the public. This opposition sets limits on what can be attempted through alcohol policy. The opposition may be weakened by a persuasive demonstration of the benefits achieved in reducing deaths and illness, but it will not disappear. Cruel as it may sound, there are other social values beyond saving lives, and we routinely make decisions that have the effect, perhaps unintended and unrecognized, of trading lives for these other values. The trade-off is quite evident in the area of traffic safety. For example, the only speed limit compatible with maximum safety is zero; and budgetary and other constraints severely limit responding to widespread opportunities to save lives by clearing roadsides of potential hazards like posts and trees and installing guardrails before bridge abutments and similar hazards.

Fortunately, the greatest benefits from alcohol seem to be maximized at relatively low BACs. The American diet is not dependent for its nutritional content on extensive alcohol consumption, and Dionysian episodes of drunkenness are looked at with ambivalence, although not necessarily total disapproval. The achievement of relaxation and enhancement of sociable interaction can be accomplished with what has been referred to as social, or normative, drinking. Although the BACs implied are associated with significant increases in the risk of serious crashes, the drunk driving problem would be greatly diminished if all higher BACs among drivers were reduced to normative levels. Alcohol policies declaring this goal, rather than abstinence, are more likely to receive general political support.

Alcohol policies as understood here are designed to reduce consumption in general or specifically in situations where driving is especially likely to occur. Most general policies—for example, those discouraging liquor advertising—can be formulated so that they pay specific attention to drunk driving, for example, by proscribing the depiction of automobiles in liquor advertisements. More restricted policies may be easier to justify as being limited to problematic drinking, and they are less likely to be opposed by interests vested in alcohol. However, general policies may be simpler to devise, and their greater reach can produce additional savings in lives by affecting the entirety of alcohol-related conditions.

The most straightforward of alcohol policies is prohibition: proscribing and penalizing the sale of alcoholic beverages. National experience with a general alcohol prohibition left this technique in disrepute, but it is currently being imposed on a limited group of young adults in the form of purchasing restrictions. Other countermeasures based in alcohol policy—price increases and restrictions on availability— attempt to affect the beverage market in order to discourage consumption. Yet another approach entails restricting advertising and promotion in order to reduce the underlying demand for alcoholic beverages. This chapter discusses the various opportunities for reducing drunk driving through alcohol policy.

Prohibition

Prohibition attempts to eliminate alcohol consumption by threatening those selling or using alcoholic beverages with criminal penalties. It terminates the legal market in the drug alcohol. The underlying premises of prohibition are that the drug is hopelessly subject to abuse and that, considering costs and benefits, society would be better off without it. It is hard to argue with these premises. Were alcohol to be introduced as a new drug, it would very likely fail to be approved by the Food and Drug Administration on the grounds that its side effects are too damaging to warrant its benefits.

This negative view of alcohol has deep roots in American history. The temperance movement, based on this view, was an important political force throughout the nineteenth century, yet it peaked at the turn of the century, before the automobile came into general use and when drunk driving was only a minor component of alcohol-related problems (Gusfield, 1963; Aaron and Musto, 1981). The temperance movement achieved enactment of the Eighteenth Amendment to the Constitution in 1919, whereby the United States joined the company of a handful of countries engaged in one of the world's most notable social experiments, dismantling the market for alcoholic beverages.

National prohibition was repealed in 1933, and since that time the conventional wisdom has been that the experiment failed. Recently, this opinion has been challenged, most notably by a panel of the National Academy of Sciences (Moore and Gerstein, 1981). If the criterion of success is the elimination of alcoholic beverages, then prohibition failed, as has virtually every countermeasure applied to any social problem. If, on the other hand, the criterion is a substantial reduction in alcohol consumption and related problems, then the experiment was successful. Consumption data from the period of national alcohol prohibition are, of course, fragmentary because true reports would frequently have involved admissions of criminal activity; but all available evidence points to a major reduction in alcohol consumption at that time. The estimate offered to the National Academy of Sciences is a decline of between a third and a half. Further, there is firm evidence of important reductions in alcohol-related crime and health statistics:

Death rates from cirrhosis were 19.5 per 100,000 in 1911 for men, and 10.7 in 1929; admissions to state mental hospital [*sic*] for disease classified as alcoholic psychosis fell from 10.1 in 1919, to 3.7 in 1922, rising to 4.7 by 1928. . . . National records of arrest for drunkenness and disorderly conduct declined 50 percent between 1916 and 1922. . . . Reports of welfare agencies from around the country over-whelmingly indicated a dramatic decrease among client population of alcohol-related family problems. [Aaron and Musto, 1981: 165]

The incomplete success of the Eighteenth Amendment and its enabling legislation, the Volstead Act, lay in the difficulty of using law to control both a simple and cheap manufacturing process and an illegal distribution process in which buyers and sellers colluded to evade the law. The legal market in alcoholic beverages was supplanted by an illegal one that sold its product at much higher prices. In consequence, while a great decrease in consumption occurred among the working classes, wealthier people were much less affected (Room, 1978). Although enforcement problems and the creation of an illegal market were important considerations in the repeal of national prohibition, the difficulties of prohibition have also been ascribed to the fact that the policy alienated important commercial interests but was unable to subdue them entirely, and it failed to develop a political and economic constituency with stakes in the new order (Aaron and Musto, 1981: 176).

The nation's disenchantment with its experience under the Eighteenth Amendment, albeit unduly extreme in light of what was accomplished, guarantees that realistic alcohol countermeasures today cannot have the breadth of a total prohibition. However, the same policy when restricted to a small segment of the population—adults aged eighteen to twenty—has been enacted into law and is having important effects on drunk driving. This policy, generally referred to as the national minimum drinking age, is actually a form of prohibition restricted to people under age twenty-one.

The national minimum drinking age

The protection of youth from avoidable harm has high priority in American policy. The death of a young person strikes us as especially tragic. The feeling can be rationalized in statistics reflecting the number of years of potential life lost when a young person dies, but this does not do justice to our grief at the loss of innocence, beauty, and other values that we associate with youth.

The largest single source of death for young people is traffic crashes, and in about half of these alcohol is present and possibly causal (Fell, 1985). Therefore, general concern about drunk driving has led to specific concern about its prevalence among young drivers. The issue of youthful drunk driving was brought to public attention by the consequences of reductions in statutory drinking ages during the 1970s. Historically, since the repeal of prohibition, most states had treated twenty-one as the age of maturity, at which point young people became entitled to the general set of rights and responsibilities conferred by adulthood. Although some capacities, such as the right to seek employment and to drive a car, were granted to much younger people, and some, such as the right to run for Congress or the presidency, were restricted to older people, twenty-one was the most significant age threshold in America. In the great majority of states, age twenty-one conferred the right to purchase and consume alcoholic beverages.

However, the "right" to military service, including that to be drafted, began at age eighteen. During the Vietnam War in the 1960s and 1970s, large numbers of people between eighteen and twenty-one served in the armed forces, voluntarily or involuntarily, and many were killed. Spokesmen for young people demanded that the obligation to fight and die for the nation be rewarded with full citizenship rights, including the right to vote, at age eighteen. This was obtained on the national level by adoption of the Twenty-sixth Amendment to the Constitution in 1971. The right to vote in state elections at age eighteen was subsequently granted in every state. In this legal environment, the restriction of drinking privileges to people over age twenty-one appeared antiquated and unjust. In most states efforts were launched to lower the legal drinking age, generally to eighteen years, and many of them were successful. Importantly, the change was not coordinated among states, which resulted in an uneven pattern of legal drinking ages across the country.

As the various states capitulated to demands to lower the drinking age, crash-related fatalities among young people began to rise, and this was interpreted by safety specialists in cause-and-effect terms. Moreover, states with higher drinking ages claimed to experience excessive numbers of crashes along borders with states having lower ages: for example, where Pennsylvania bordered New York and Illinois bordered Wisconsin. Although the existence of a border problem has not been confirmed in research, the general association of lower drinking ages with higher numbers of crashes in the newly enfranchised age group was repeatedly demonstrated (Wagenaar, 1983).

The crash-fatality evidence was sufficiently convincing that some states retracted their recent grants of freedom to drink at ages under twenty-one. Between 1976 and 1980, eleven states raised their minimum drinking ages from eighteen to nineteen, twenty, or twenty-one. Michigan, for instance, which had reduced the minimum drinking age to eighteen in 1972, raised it to twenty-one in December 1978. Initial evaluations (e.g., Wagenaar, 1981; Williams et al., 1983) gave hope that higher minimum drinking ages would be rewarded with fewer alcohol-involved crashes. The idea of a uniform national minimum drinking age of twenty-one years began to be discussed in the safety community, including the National Transportation Safety Board and the National Highway Traffic Safety Administration, and in the deliberations of the Presidential Commission on Drunk Driving. This evidence helped convince the presidential commission (1983) to recommend that all states adopt twenty-one as the minimum drinking age. The Reagan administration, along with many of the commission members, was generally uncomfortable with federal action in a field traditionally allocated to the states. However, the difficulty of dealing by means of state and local action with the presumed border problems helped achieve the administration's endorsement. Legislation passed in 1984 encouraged states to enact the twenty-one-year drinking age by threatening to withhold federal highway construction funds from those not complying. Although the requirement encountered considerable resistance, including a constitutional challenge by South Dakota, all states eventually complied.

The twenty-one-year national minimum drinking age is one of the most thoroughly evaluated social interventions of our time. The evaluation literature has been summarized by the General Accounting Office (GAO) (1987). Overall, this review of forty-nine studies of raised drinking ages found strong evidence of its effectiveness. The GAO report concluded,

Raising the drinking age has a direct effect on reducing alcohol-related traffic accidents among youths affected by the laws. The evidence also supports the finding that states can generally expect reductions in their [total] traffic accidents, but the magnitude of the effects depends on the outcome measured and the characteristics of the state. The available evidence suggests that raising the drinking age also results in a decline in alcohol consumption and in driving after drinking for the age group affected by the law. . . .

The evidence is insufficient to draw conclusions about the effects of raising the drinking age on youths 16 to 17 years old, border crossings, and other related matters. However, the literature reviews of earlier evaluations of the effects of *lowering* the drinking age do give evidence that traffic-accident outcomes increased as a result of changes in the law. [1987: 3]

In research completed after the GAO review was published, Wagenaar and O'Malley (1990) determined on the basis of self-reports of drinking behavior that the reduction in drinking among those under the new legal age continues to some extent as young adults mature beyond the legal drinking age. Furthermore, this reduction, although modest in size, is concentrated in the consumption in bars and taverns, that is, drinking frequently associated with driving. Drinking in cars does not appear to have increased, as some people feared.

The success of the national minimum drinking age symbolizes the ability of prohibition legislation to contain alcohol-related problems. However, this form of prohibition, like the broader one of the 1920s, works in a far from perfect manner. Young people still drink. A national survey conducted in 1989, when the drinking age was twenty-one in all states, demonstrates this. It found that 60 percent of high school seniors reported having drunk alcohol during the previous month, and 33 percent had at least one occasion of heavy drinking (five or more drinks in a row) in the previous two weeks (National Commission on Drug-Free Schools, 1990: 64). Moreover, much of the drinking of young people is heavy, or binge, drinking: about half of the first-year college students studied by Wechsler and Isaac (1991) usually drank five or more drinks on a single occasion. More than half the men and more than a third of the women reported such an occasion within the previous two weeks. Much of this drinking was in association with driving. For instance, 37 percent of high school seniors in a Pennsylvania county reported having driven after drinking (or taking drugs) during the previous six months (Strand and Garr, 1990). The study of Boston-area first-year college students (Wechsler and Isaac, 1991) reported such behavior for more than half the men and more than a third of the women during the previous year.

A senior official of a major brewing company, in an interview in 1984 concerning the presidential commission's recommendations, told me his company's estimate: Were all young people in states with drinking ages lower than twenty-one to cease consuming beer, the company's market would diminish by 7 percent. However, the estimate of actual impact, based on experience with states that had previously raised the drinking age, was a market loss of only 2 percent.

The National Institute on Alcohol Abuse and Alcoholism (1990: 217) also noted the imperfect functioning of minimum drinking-age laws: "Although changes in the laws regulating minimum drinking age may have had some effect on consumption, they have not eliminated access to alcohol nor deterred many adolescents from drinking."

That minimum drinking-age laws should operate imperfectly might be expected, given the existence of a legal market in alcoholic beverages for people over twenty-one and the lack of any social, much less physical, segregation of people over and under the critical age. Wagenaar and O'Malley offer the following explanation for the limited ability of drinking-age laws to control drinking among high school students:

> The popularity of drinking among seniors is not surprising. Alcohol use is a very common social practice among adults, particularly among young adults, and that alone would tend to make it an attractive activity for adolescents. And enforcement of minimum drinking age laws tends to be lax in most states. In addition, the use of alcohol is heavily promoted and glamorized in commercials; the entire aura around those commercials is pleasurable, athletic, sexual, fun—all the things that appeal to youth. Consequently, many more societal changes are needed in addition to changes in minimum drinking age laws if drinking among high school seniors is to be further reduced. [1990: 26]

The claim of lax enforcement is supported by a study of the Insurance Institute for Highway Safety (Preusser and Williams, 1991) in which young men aged nineteen and twenty were sent to buy beer in a variety of stores in Washington, D.C., and two sites in New York State. They succeeded in 97 percent of attempts in Washington, and 80 percent of attempts in Westchester County, New York. They were successful only

44 percent of the time in Albany and Schenectady. In these cities, recent police enforcement of purchase age laws may have affected the behavior of the sellers.

All countermeasures are partial and imperfect, however. Most observers would agree that measures reducing fatalities by 9 percent (the estimate of DuMouchel, Williams, and Zador, 1987) or even as much as 18 percent (the estimate of Saffer and Grossman, 1987a) would represent important progress in saving lives. DuMouchel, Williams, and Zador estimated that as a result of increases in the legal drinking age in twenty-six states between 1975 and 1984, 370 young men and 216 young women had avoided premature deaths. The National Highway Traffic Safety Administration estimates that more than 10,000 youthful lives have been saved because of adoptions of twenty-one (National Center for Statistics and Analysis, 1990). Grossman (1988) points to 555 youthful lives that could have been saved each year if the twenty-one-year drinking age had prevailed nationally in the period 1975–81. The effect of drinking-age laws may be amplified through the passage of laws that lower the tolerated BAC for young drivers (Hingson et al., 1990). In all events, the minimum drinking age appears to have helped create an environment supportive of related countermeasures, such as alcohol-free schools and colleges. It legitimizes their goals and reduces the opportunities to violate their rules.

It is possible to argue that prohibition is a costly and unjust approach to reducing drunk driving. As the alcohol industry stresses, most drinkers do not encounter alcohol-related problems, yet the privileges of all are curtailed by prohibitionist countermeasures. What is more, limiting the prohibition to a group which, although from one perspective disproportionately involved in drunk driving, constitutes only a fraction of the problem (Fell, 1987) may produce the impression that matters are under control, while the rest of the population remains free to continue engaging in activity that produces the bulk of the problem. Indeed, the highest proportion of alcohol-related fatalities is not among teenagers, but rather among those aged twenty-five to twenty-nine, whose right to drink is unquestioned (National Highway Traffic Safety Administration, 1991).

It is no longer possible to argue that prohibition can't work as a policy to save lives. The national minimum drinking age is effective in reducing alcohol consumption among the group to which it applies, and the effect persists for a cohort even after they graduate to ages at which drinking is legal. It can be seen not only as fulfilling the promise of prohibition, but as a validation of the general principle of alcohol-based countermeasures, namely, that reducing total alcohol consumption can reduce alcohol-related problems. Its success is based on its potential to alter one of the fundamental institutional causes of drunk driving.

Market control mechanisms

Market interventions postulate that increasing the price and decreasing the availability of alcoholic beverages will reduce consumption and thus reduce alcohol-related problems. They assume an existing market for alcoholic beverages that is legal but that externalizes many of the costs associated with consumption of the product.

Market mechanisms have numerous advantages over criminal-justice approaches to alcohol problems. Perhaps the most obvious is that they appear noncoercive. Instead of criminal proscriptions, the market offers disincentives, which seem external and impersonal, retaining for the individual the opportunity to choose the discouraged option and pay its price. Morality, which is at the heart of the criminal law, is irrelevant. While the market may dissuade, it neither condemns nor demands vengeance.

Market mechanisms, by avoiding concern with reform and rehabilitation, accept people as they are. Choices judged inappropriate by policymakers are handled by making it more difficult to act upon them; no attempt is made to change personalities, motives, and instincts.

A major barrier to the use of market mechanisms can be the ability of people to circumvent the constrained legal market through recourse to an illegal one. This occurred on a grand scale during national prohibition, and it appears to have importantly reduced the benefits theoretically attainable from recent increases in the legal drinking age. However, the costs of establishing and defending illegal markets permit some manipulation of legal ones without the experience of serious challenges. Furthermore, the examples just reviewed show that some of the goals of market control can be achieved even in the presence of extensive evasions.

An indirect relationship between consumption of a commodity and consequent social problems furnishes another caution against relying on market mechanisms to reduce the problems. Broad and undifferentiated measures like price increases due to taxation can reduce consumption of a product, but the related problem may not be controlled to the same degree. Some problems are directly related to the amount of alcohol consumed, but other problems are linked less directly. For these, the reasonableness of market manipulation requires investigation and demonstration. Cirrhosis of the liver is in the former category; it is a fairly straightforward consequence of the total amount of alcohol consumed over a drinker's lifetime (Cook and Tauchen, 1982). Many other problems are related not just to the amount consumed, but to the manner of consumption and its consequent impact on BAC. Violent behavior, including drunk driving, is of this type. Additionally, the circumstances of consumption—the time and place and social setting—may be of crucial importance. Reduced consumption at Sunday Communion ceremonies, for example, is of little policy importance, whereas reducing drinking at rowdy roadhouses would be an appropriate target for countermeasures. To devise market constraints that more strongly affect dangerous kinds of consumption is a major challenge. However, since the vast bulk of drinking has negative consequences for traffic safety by raising crash risk to some degree, the use of broad, unspecific market controls is an acceptable approach from the viewpoint of saving lives.

Market mechanisms can be divided into the categories of pricing and availability constraints. The price of alcoholic beverages can be increased by imposing special taxes on them. Their availability can be restricted by more stringent regulations than apply to consumer goods in general. Considerable research on both topics supports the proposition that these mechanisms can reduce drunk driving.

Pricing

Pricing countermeasures proceed from the assumption that alcohol consumption, like that of nearly all commodities, decreases as its price rises. The relationship between price and consumption is described by means of the concept of elasticity in economics. This refers to the amount of change in consumption of a commodity as a result of a change in price or other factors (Ornstein and Levy, 1983: 305). Price elasticity is typically negative, that is, the higher the price, the less consumed. Consumption of a commodity with a price elasticity of -0.5 is expected to decline by 5 percent for every 10 percent increase in price. A commodity with an elasticity of -1.0 would decline percentagewise in consumption in the same amount as the percentage increase in price. If purchasers are determined to have a commodity, its price elasticity will be low; if consumers consider it a dispensable frill, price elasticity will be high. Consumption is also elastic with regard to income, and this relation is usually positive: the higher the purchaser's income, the more of the commodity is consumed.

Models of Markets Two general theoretical models of the market for alcoholic beverages are relevant to the ability of price increases to reduce alcohol-related problems. One of these, termed unimodal or constant proportion (Room, 1978), asserts that all consumption is a function of the average amount consumed. The higher this average, the more drinks will be consumed by all parts of the population, and the lower this average, the less will be consumed by all. To the extent that this model describes the market accurately, it follows that price increases will reduce drinking by all kinds of consumers and, doubtless, have an important impact on drunk driving.

A contrasting conceptualization asserts the existence of different types of consumers with different price elasticities. This model, termed bimodal, envisages one group of ordinary drinkers, whose consumption follows the norm, dropping as prices increase, and another group of determined drinkers—problem drinkers, alcoholics, and addicts— whose demand is insistent and who will drink a great deal regardless of price. To the extent that this model describes the population, the impact of price increases on drunk driving will be very much reduced, since they are expected to have less effect on those who drink the most heavily and engage in the most impaired driving.

Much debate in the field of alcohol research has focused on whether a specific variant of the unimodal model, termed the Ledermann curve, is supported by empirical evidence. As Room (1984) points out, this narrow question has little importance. The bulk of research in numerous countries supports the unimodal model along with the corollary that even the most confirmed drinkers respond to the price of alcohol (Ahlstrom, 1983; Single, 1991). This view, strongly endorsed by the Finnish Foundation for Alcohol Studies and the Addiction Research Foundation of Ontario (Mäkelä et al., 1981), clearly prevailed in the deliberations of the National Academy of Science's Transportation Research Board (Moore and Gerstein, 1981) and in the Surgeon General's Workshop on Drunk Driving (Wagenaar and Farrell, 1989). According to these authorities, it can be confidently asserted on theoretical and empirical bases that raising the price of alcoholic beverages will diminish consumption in some degree by all kinds of drinkers, including the heaviest consumers, and that this reduces the occurrence of alcohol-related problems, including drunk driving.

The role of taxes The price of alcoholic beverages can be raised through excise tax increases. A tax increase may not raise consumer prices to the same extent—for example, producers or distributors may choose to bear some or all of the tax, resulting in price changes less than the tax; alternatively, retailers may apply markups to a tax as well as to the basic cost of the product, resulting in price increases greater than the tax increase. However, significant alcohol tax increases can generally be expected to result in some increase in prices to consumers, and to the degree that consumption is elastic, consumption of alcohol will be reduced. To the degree that alcohol problems, including drunk driving, are responsive to changes in consumption, they will also be reduced.

Taxation for the purpose of raising the price and reducing consumption of a problematic commodity has to be distinguished from that undertaken to gain revenue. The optimal tax from the latter viewpoint is that which raises the most money. From the viewpoint of discouraging consumption, the optimal tax is generally much higher and total revenues are disproportionally lowered because of decreased purchases. Many economists specify the optimum as the point at which tax revenues equal the total costs attributable to alcohol less the benefits experienced from drinking (Phelps, 1988; Manning et al., 1989). At this point, the market price of alcoholic beverages fully reflects the net social costs of alcohol-related problems. This can be regarded as a theoretical limit on tax policy. Tax policy is also pragmatically limited by public tolerance and the potential for evasion.

From the viewpoint of taxing to limit consumption, the purposes to which the tax money is put are largely irrelevant. Alcohol taxes are nonetheless often tied to programs directed at treating alcohol-related problems. The tie may help sell a tax increase by generating support from vested interests. For instance, a tax tied to therapeutic programs may be vigorously supported by physicians and psychologists. Its main danger lies in the diversion of attention from consumption per se. The tie implies that the tax is sufficiently high if it covers the costs of the tied programs, whereas this level may be far from optimal for lowering consumption.

The opportunity to reduce alcohol-related problems, including drunk driving, through taxation has been considerably overlooked in recent years. In historical context as well as in comparison with other countries the principal taxes on alcoholic beverages in the United States today— those imposed by the federal government—are insignificant. They are also irrational from the viewpoint of discouraging alcohol consumption because they favor some sources of alcohol over others even though the impairing effect of a given quantity of the drug varies little with the type of beverage in which it is contained.

In contrast to the present-day situation, alcohol taxes were very important in the past. As recently as the first decade of the twentieth century, they accounted for 80 percent of all federal revenues. Their decline in importance is reflected in the fact that in 1984 they accounted for a mere 1 percent of such revenues in the United States, as compared, for example, with 22 percent in Poland, 5 to 6 percent in Denmark, Britain, Hungary, and Ireland, and 2 to 3 percent in Canada, Japan, Australia, and Spain (National Alcohol Tax Coalition, 1989: 3).

Following the repeal of national prohibition, taxes on alcoholic beverages were kept low because lawmakers feared that high taxes might create an illegal market. The federal excise tax was set at $2.00 per gallon of 100 proof distilled spirits, 16 cents per gallon of beer, and 10 cents per gallon of wine. The tax per ounce of alcohol in beer and wine was much lower than for spirits on the theory that consumption of these "moderate" beverages should be encouraged. This theory is now discredited, especially by the knowledge that beer is the drunk driver's beverage of choice (Berger and Snortum, 1985; Greenfeld, 1988).

Federal alcohol excise taxes were modestly raised over the years until 1951, when they were set at $10.50 for spirits, 29 cents for beer, and 17 cents for wine. In 1985 the rate on spirits was increased to $12.50, while the other taxes remained as before until 1990. The 1951 taxes became deeply discounted by subsequent inflation. Between 1951 and 1985 the value of the dollar, and thus of the excise taxes, declined by 75 percent. This was modestly compensated for by the 19 percent increase in the spirits tax in 1985, but there was no tax increase on beer and wine. This decline in the absolute level of taxation was an important factor in keeping the real price of alcoholic beverages low. Between 1967 and 1987 the price of liquor in constant dollars declined by 50 percent, and the price of beer and wine (in which taxes are a less important factor) declined by 28 percent (National Alcohol Tax Coalition 1989: 4, citing congressional testimony by Philip Cook). In 1990, the federal tax on a 1.4-ounce glass of 80-proof liquor was 11 cents; that on a 12-ounce beer with about the same amount of alcohol was less than 3 cents; and that on a 4.7-ounce glass of wine, again with comparable alcohol, was less than 1 cent. Although state excise taxes added to their cost, it was a matter of common notice that alcoholic beverages had become extraordinarily cheap in the United States and particularly that beer was often cheaper than soda.

Legislation passed in 1990 raised the federal tax on alcohol, but it fell far short of fully compensating for inflation since 1951 or fully equalizing the tax among beverages according to their alcohol content. Had the tax on spirits been recalculated to account for inflation, it would have been about $40 per 100-proof gallon. The actual tax on spirits was increased by 8 percent, to $13.50 per 100-proof gallon, or about 12 cents per standard drink. That on beer was doubled, to the equivalent of 32 cents per six-pack, and that on wine increased sixfold, to the equivalent of about 21 cents per bottle. Fiscal concerns combined with health ones to raise the tax, along with that on cigarettes, but alcohol industry lobbyists kept the increase far lower than what public health spokespersons had proposed. Indeed, the tax increases recommended by the Surgeon General's Workshop on Drunk Driving in 1988 would have raised eight times as much revenue as those actually adopted by Congress in 1990 (Center for Science in the Public Interest, 1990).

Clearly the federal alcohol excise taxes of 1990 added relatively little to the cost of alcohol over what it might have been in the absence of tax, and the increases were modest in comparison to the consequences of returning taxes to the contemporary equivalent of 1951 levels. The significance of the reference to 1951 is that there was no important illegal market in alcohol at that time, which suggests that taxes at the level of 1951 very likely would be tolerable today. Thus, it seems that a tax in 1990 dollars of about $40 per gallon of spirits—about 35 cents per drink—which might have a major impact on alcohol consumption and alcohol problems, would not likely be accompanied by prohibition-style illegal production and black markets.

Consequences of tax policies The actual reduction in alcohol consumption and related problems achieved from tax increases has generated a considerable international economic literature. It is fair to say that few scholars doubt that a major tax increase would significantly reduce alcohol consumption and related problems, but estimates of the amount of reduction vary considerably. One way of stating the issue is to say that researchers vary in their estimates of the price elasticity of alcohol.

The early literature on this topic (summarized by Ornstein and Levy, 1983) has been buttressed by recent research on the effect of alcohol taxes on drunk driving. Important American studies on drunk driving include Cook on the consequences of state increases in the liquor tax (1981; Cook and Tauchen, 1982); Saffer and Grossman (1987a; 1987b) on the impact of the beer tax on young drivers; and Phelps (1988), who used survey data relevant to demand for alcoholic beverages. Cook estimated that a 10 percent increase in the price of liquor would result in a 7 percent decrease in crash-related fatalities. Saffer and Grossman estimated that a doubling of the beer tax would reduce highway deaths 18 percent among youths aged fifteen to seventeen, 27 percent among those eighteen to twenty, and 19 percent among those twenty-one to twenty-four. Phelps estimated that a 10 percent increase in the beer tax would result in a 12 percent decline in fatalities.

These studies met with considerable criticism, not only because of the inherent imprecision of estimates obtained by econometric modeling, but also because of the impact on the policy debate of some extrapolations that went far beyond the available data. For example, Saffer and Grossman suggested that tax policy would be more successful in reducing youthful deaths than drinking-age policy. They calculated that a tax rate resulting from the equalizing of beer and wine taxes with that on spirits and from indexing for inflation from 1951 would have reduced crash fatalities among young people by more than half. This is a far greater reduction than that accomplished by the imposition of the national minimum drinking age of twenty-one. (It may have been unwise for the authors to offer this striking extrapolation from their analysis, as it was justifiably used by critics to impeach the model's assumptions.)

In my opinion, although the methodological problems inherent in these studies can cast doubt on specific price-elasticity estimates and therefore on specific projections of impact for tax policy, the consistency of findings and their alignment with theory supports the view that substantial increases in alcohol taxes offer an important opportunity to save lives. This conclusion parallels that of the Panel on Pricing and Availability in the Surgeon General's Workshop on Drunk Driving (Office of the Surgeon General, 1989: 18): "Research evidence shows that an increase in the excise tax could have the largest long-term effect on alcohol-impaired driving of all policy and program options available."

Optimal taxation How high should alcohol taxes be? Economists may answer this question by estimating externalized costs (those not included in the price of alcohol by the unregulated market) and proposing taxes to cover them (Manning et al., 1989). The bulk of these externalized costs consists of the value of lives lost in alcohol-related crashes, and differences in this valuation can result in huge discrepancies in the estimated costs and proposed taxes. The figure used by Manning et al., $1.66 million per life, was extrapolated from evidence of people's willingness to pay for small chances of surviving. The figure is arguable, not only because of questions concerning the legitimacy of the extrapolation; for example, it does not include expenses incurred by surviving nondrinking victims of crashes caused by alcohol, yet it includes costs of lives lost in crashes in which alcohol was present but may not have been a causal factor. If the figures are accepted as an approximation, however, the bottom-line best estimate of social cost can be calculated as $1.19 for each "excessive" ounce of alcohol (defined as anything over two drinks per day).

Manning et al. confess to having disregarded several economically significant factors that might be taken into account in setting the alcohol tax, including issues such as the impact of addiction on demand and the limits of consumer information. Although, as noted, the assumptions on which this estimate is based are contestable and imprecise, Phelps, using somewhat different methods, has also estimated optimal tax levels for alcohol and endorsed a large increase (1988: 206). It appears that the true optimum tax, whatever it might be, is most likely much higher than what is now politically feasible. In other words, proponents of an alcohol tax that stands a reasonable chance of being passed by a legislature probably need not be concerned that it exceeds the economic optimum.

A final consideration about taxation is that it may be desirable to impose higher rates, and thereby more steeply discourage consumption, in situations in which subsequent driving is especially likely. This cannot be done with pinpoint accuracy, but research has identified establishments that sell alcohol for on-premise consumption (bars and taverns) as a class of outlets especially involved with drunk driving. O'Donnell's (1985) review of eleven studies of this subject found such premises to be the drinking place of 40 to 63 percent of drivers arrested for drunk driving, 43 to 64 percent of drivers with BACs over 0.10 percent in roadside surveys, and 26 percent of drivers involved in alcohol-related crashes: "People tend to go to bars to continue the drinking they started elsewhere; bars appear to be a site for heavy drinking; and more people may drive away from bars in an intoxicated state than from other drinking locations" (1985: 515).

An even greater incidence of bar drinking among the most problematic drunk drivers was found in more recent research (Wieczorek, Miller, and Nochajski, 1989). Among arrested drunk drivers referred to the Drinking Driver Treatment and Evaluation Program in Erie County (Buffalo), New York, because of high alcoholism screening scores, high BACs, or multiple offenses, 69 percent mentioned drinking in bars prior to arrest. This contrasted with 10 percent drinking at home, 20 percent in someone else's home, and only 5 percent in restaurants. (Some persons drank at more than one place, so percentages add to more than 100.)

In addition, some case studies of bars have found that large fractions of patrons leave licensed premises with illegal BACs. Even when presented with the results of breath tests and being told that it is illegal to drive with a BAC above the legal limit, the vast majority of over-the-limit patrons drive off (Van Houten, Nau, and Jonah, 1983; Meier, Brigham, and Handel, 1984).

This evidence suggests an opportunity for reducing drunk driving through server intervention and other control policies instituted in bars and taverns; these will be discussed below. For the present topic of taxation, the evidence justifies the imposition of surtaxes on alcoholic beverages served in these locations. Although some consumers will doubtless decide to shift their drinking from bars to other locations, it is likely that total consumption will be reduced and that the alternative locations will involve less driving after drinking.

Taxes: conclusion Increasing the price of alcohol, like raising the legal drinking age, impacts some elements of the population more than others. On that ground, its fairness can be questioned. For both measures, however, it can be argued that those who pay the cost are also disproportionately the beneficiaries, in that they avoid injuries and premature death. Moreover, those who disapprove of the regressive burdens of alcohol taxation can obviate such an effect by progressively shifting the overall tax system so that economically disadvantaged drinkers are no more highly taxed than advantaged ones.

Raising the price of alcoholic beverages offers an important opportunity for reducing drunk driving. An increase in taxes seems called for on the basis that lives can be saved through policy that seems economically advisable and politically feasible. Although this action receives additional support and justification to the extent that tax revenues are targeted for education and treatment programs, the price increase is justifiable in and of itself, since it serves to reduce alcohol consumption and consequent problems. Such taxation has been recommended by policy groups of both liberal (National Alcohol Tax Coalition, 1989) and conservative (National Commission on Drug-Free Schools, 1990) persuasions. In addition, ample poll data show that two-thirds to three-quarters of the public supports the principle of raising alcohol taxes, not just to balance budgets or fund treatment, but, as respondents in, respectively, Minnesota (Armson, 1990) and Michigan (Wagenaar et al., 1988) stated, "to reduce drunk driving" and "to rid the . . . roadways of alcohol-impaired drivers." Although the failure of proposals to increase alcohol taxes in state elections in 1990 suggests that this support may be shallow, the superficially favorable attitude toward alcohol tax increases may be deepened by further demonstrations of the extent of alcohol-related problems and the reasonableness of the belief that tax increases can affect these.

Availability constraints

A second category of market controls is reductions in availability. This approach is related to pricing, in that both constrain our ability to purchase alcoholic beverages. Contemplation of either can reduce consumption, just as both long lines and high prices can reduce our interest in going to the movies on a Saturday night. Availability constraints include limits on the numbers of establishments selling alcoholic beverages, both in general and with reference to types disproportionately involved in creating drunk driving. Other constraints limit service locations and hours of operation.

The numbers of sales outlets There is considerable research on the proposition that numbers of sales outlets correlate with alcohol consumption. The best and most relevant data come from Scandinavia, where previously tight controls on availability have been relaxed in recent years. The Finnish experience is particularly interesting, offering examples of such innovations as placing liquor stores in rural communities, permitting expansion of the numbers of so-called restaurants serving alcohol, and allowing the sale of moderately strong beer in food stores (Mäkelä, Österberg, and Sulkunen, 1981). Relevant American experiences include the privatization of wine sales in certain monopoly states (Wagenaar and Holder, 1990) and permission for restaurants to sell liquor by the drink (Blose and Holder 1987a; Holder and Blose, 1987). Differential alcohol availability within the United States also permits cross-sectional analyses of the relationship between the distribution pattern and alcohol consumption and problems (Rabow and Watts, 1982; Hooper, 1983; Colon, 1983; Colon and Cutter, 1982).

This literature generally supports the proposition that the greater the numbers of opportunities to purchase alcohol, the greater the consumption (Macdonald and Whitehead, 1983). However, there have been exceptions. Smart (1977), for instance, found that income and urbanism were more closely related to consumption and reported alcoholism than was an index of availability of alcoholic beverages (see also Neuman and Rabow, 1986). Increases in reported total consumption have sometimes been accompanied by declines in estimated illegal consumption, so that changes in legal sales may overstate the effects of liberalized control policies (Horverak, 1989). The studies by Blose and Holder found that liquor consumed legally by the drink largely replaced previous legal—and less expensive—brown-bagging by restaurant customers, which presents similar cautions for interpreting the results.

Of more direct concern is the relationship between numbers of outlets and alcohol-related problems, especially drunk driving. Here, the literature gives mixed signals. Fewer outlets are associated with fewer of the kinds of problems most directly related to consumption, such as cirrhosis (Hooper, 1983; Rush, Gliksman, and Brook, 1986; Rabow and Watts, 1982). A similar association has been reported in some studies of drunk driving. For example, Rabow and Watts found that the numbers of retail liquor outlets correlate with drunk driving arrests. Blose and Holder (1987b) found adoption of liquor-by-the-drink in North Carolina to be associated with increases in alcohol-related crashes (a weak index, owing to variations in police records) and with single-vehicle nighttime crashes involving males of drinking age.

In contrast, the work of Colon and other investigators finds that, although average beer consumption is positively related to highway fatalities, the combination of counties prohibiting the sale of alcohol (dry counties) in proximity to counties permitting it (wet counties) apparently produces more alcohol-related fatalities than does uniform permissiveness. This holds even though the uniformly permissive jurisdictions presumably have more liquor outlets. Indeed, the counties without legal alcohol sales have higher motor-vehicle fatality rates than the wet counties:

> Had the rates been the same it might be argued that restrictive measures, such as prohibition, at least serve symbolic ends. These results, however, demonstrate that such measures can exacerbate the very conditions they were designed to remedy. . . .
>
> A tentative hypothesis suggested by the data is that drinkers in dry counties drive to neighboring counties and states to purchase alcoholic beverages. They thereby increase their accident risk through added driving and through driving under the influence when purchases are made in taverns. [Colon, 1983: 103–04]

Colon's conclusion concerning these data has been challenged by Joksch (1991), who notes that there is no relationship between traffic fatalities and the proportion of the population living in dry counties. Such a relationship would be expected on the basis of Colon's need-to-drive hypothesis.

A study of Tennessee cities with differing liquor laws found an inverse relationship between the permissiveness of legislation and alcohol problem indexes, including motor vehicle fatalities (Dull and Giacopassi, 1986). Likewise, some studies of adoption of liquor-by-the-drink found no effect on crashes, and one study even reported a decrease (Speiglman and Goetz, 1987).

Briefly, the extent of drunk driving does not appear to be a simple function of numbers of outlets, possibly because the purchase of alcohol in some kinds of outlets is less likely to be associated with driving; it may even reduce the amount of driving that might otherwise take place. This suggests the need to attend to the characteristics of alcohol outlets as factors in producing drunk driving.

Types of outlets We may speculate that the most dangerous form of alcohol consumption from the viewpoint of drunk driving is that which occurs in cars. For instance, a study of drivers arrested for driving under the influence in San Diego found that more than half had consumed alcohol in their cars shortly after purchasing it from liquor stores, convenience stores, or gasoline station minimarts (Segars and Ryan, 1986; Wittman, 1986).

Some kinds of sales outlets may encourage drinking in cars, at least symbolically, by supporting an image of alcohol and driving as being compatible; they may encourage it materially as well. Two such types of outlets are stores that sell to vehicle occupants through drive-up windows and gasoline stations that sell alcoholic beverages. There is no competent research on the effect of drive-up windows, and there is little on gasoline station sales. The study of arrested drunk drivers in San Diego found that the ratio of drinking episodes in cars to the amount of alcohol purchased was highest for outlets that sold both alcohol and gasoline. The car-drinking rate for beverages purchased at gas stations was nearly three times as high as for alcohol purchases overall. However, only 6 percent of the outlets patronized by the drunk drivers were of this type, and the bulk of in-car drinking followed purchases from liquor stores and convenience stores. A study in Sonoma County, California, found that only 2 percent of drunk drivers in that jurisdiction had purchased their beverages from so-called gasmarts (Fontaine, 1992).

Although the evidence is thin, it does suggest that proliferation of gasoline stations that sell alcoholic beverages could result in increases in drunk driving, and conversely that drunk driving might be reduced by prohibiting the sale of automobile fuels and alcoholic beverages on the same premises. In addition, although no scientific evidence is available, there would seem to be little social benefit, and some possible harm, from permitting liquor stores to serve through drive-up windows. Not only is the conjunction of drinking and driving symbolized and facilitated in these outlets, but one may speculate that drinking-age and service-to-intoxicated laws are more easily evaded in such facilities. As Wittmann (1986) points out, regulations restricting alcohol sales in gasoline stations and through drive-up windows could be enacted in local legislation based on zoning and similar powers as well as by formal liquor control laws, which are usually part of state codes. Given the lack of present scientific evidence of effectiveness for these counter-measures, it is important that legislation enacting them contain pro-visions for their evaluation.

If prohibition of sales of alcoholic beverages in close conjunction with the automobile were judged too extreme a measure, a more moderate intervention would require that the beverages sold for off-premise consumption not be ready for immediate drinking, that is, that beer and wine be sold unchilled and that spirits be sold unmixed. The beverages would of course remain drinkable and the alcohol in them just as intoxicating, but the lack of palatability might help to weaken the association of these sales with immediate consumption in auto-mobiles. Passage of open container laws aimed at deterring drinking in vehicles might be a useful adjunct to efforts to separate drinking from driving. Such laws are symbolically appropriate in indicating the unacceptability of drinking in cars, although again there is no scientific evidence concerning their effectiveness in reducing drunk driving.

The most important source of drunk drivers, according to numerous surveys, is bars and taverns. As noted above, about half of surveyed drivers with illegal BACs report having drunk in licensed premises, and in studies distinguishing bars from restaurants and other licensed sites it is the bars that are most heavily involved in creating drunk drivers (O'Donnell, 1985: 15). Countermeasures that address the norms and practices of beverage service in bars will be discussed below. Here, it is suggested that proliferation of on-premise consumption outlets may be especially likely to increase drunk driving, and thus that limits to this proliferation are likely to save lives. However, as suggested by Colon (1982), below certain outlet densities the need to drive in order to reach the drinking destination could paradoxically result in fewer bars producing more drunk driving. Caution regarding recommendations for stringent limits on alcohol outlets is also war-ranted by the findings of Dull and Giacopassi (1986) reported above and of Macdonald and Whitehead (1983), who, although finding persuasive evidence of a relationship between alcohol consumption and numbers of off-premise outlets (liquor stores), did not find one with on-premise outlets.

Locations and hours The possibility of controlling the location of alcoholic beverage outlets in order to reduce drunk driving is an intriguing research issue. At present, little is known because few jurisdictions have developed relevant policies. Governments commonly prohibit alcohol sales in proximity to churches and schools in the United States, but I know of no examples of prohibiting such sales in proximity to highways, for instance. Highway locations are in fact common among establishments offering on-premise consumption of alcoholic beverages, and governments may inadvertently help assure that drinkers arrive and leave by car through the requirement that such establishments provide adequate parking. There has been relatively little questioning of the view that bars are acceptable roadside businesses, just like food shops, motels, and gasoline stations.

Although research on the effects of these arrangements is lacking, situating bars in the vicinity of highways appears intuitively to give wrong messages concerning the association of drinking and driving. Such messages could be avoided by discouraging highway locations for drinking establishments through zoning and by fees related to the number of adjacent parking spaces. Similar reasoning leads to the (possibly unnecessary) recommendation that governments not permit the sale of alcoholic beverages in such locations as service areas on turnpikes.

Although the location of drinking establishments with respect to highways has not been addressed in existing liquor control policy, restrictions on licensed-premises service hours have prevailed widely, and they are often justified as means of controlling drinking. However, existing research does not give much reason to expect drunk driving reductions from this type of regulation. Reduced hours for selling alcohol were found to be associated with reductions in alcohol-related problems in some Scandinavian studies (Room, 1984: 310), but lengthening of sales hours did not necessarily increase them. It has been argued even that longer drinking hours may reduce the pressure to drink heavily and therefore reduce drunk driving (Association of Erie County Liquor Licensees, n.d.). Evidence from an important shift in closing times—from 6 P.M. to 10 P.M.—in the state of Victoria in Australia provides no firm answer. Although the peak hour for crashes predictably shifted, the numbers of crashes were not significantly changed (Birrell, 1975). Likewise, the liberalization of opening hours for pubs in Scotland was not associated with diminished highway safety (Ashley and Rankin, 1988).

What seems intuitively obvious is that differentials in closing hours among neighboring jurisdictions furnish incentives to drive after drinking. This is like the border problem noted for different drinking ages before the national minimum was instituted, only it is related to time differences rather than age differences. Since closing hours are often matters of local rather than state law, the opportunities for them to differ are considerable; removing such differences would appear to be sensible policy. Unfortunately, no good evidence is currently available concerning safety benefits to be derived from uniform closing hours.

Availability: conclusion In sum, it appears that restrictions on the availability of alcoholic beverages—especially controls over the numbers and types of sales outlets—may under some circumstances reduce alcohol consumption and related problems. However, the relationship between outlets and alcohol problems is not a simple one, and in some situations more outlets appear to result in less drunk driving. The evidence for benefits from restricting locations and hours is mainly intuitive. Although policies based on these principles convey appropriate symbols and may contribute to a desirable long-run general change in the role of alcohol in society, it is not reasonable to look to them for major short-run accomplishments (Room, 1984; Hauge, 1988). Indeed, excessive restrictions on hours and sales locations may be ineffective in reducing alcohol consumption and related problems, and these might be abandoned without a loss of safety. Measures enacted to restrict alcohol availability in order to reduce drunk driving should be endorsed only provisionally and should be subjected to thorough evaluation.

Constraints on service

The fact that licensed premises are important as origins of drunk drivers found on the highways raises the possibility of placing constraints on service practices as possible drunk driving countermeasures. The role of bars in creating drunk driving is explained by the fact that people drive to and from them in order to drink, and they drink relatively heavily in many bar environments once they arrive. The Buffalo study of drunk drivers noted, "Bar drinkers and home drinkers appear to possess different drinking styles. Bar drinkers consumed more alcohol immediately prior to their arrest... and reported drinking more alcohol per occasion" (Wieczorek, Miller, and Nochajski, 1989). Large segments of departing clientele have been noted to achieve BACs that would be illegal were they to drive, and the great majority are significantly impaired as drivers (e.g., Russ and Geller, 1987; Meier, Brigham, and Handel, 1984; Van Houten, Nau, and Jonah, 1983). That they get into their cars and drive off is virtually guaranteed by the spatial structure of American communities.

Indeed, drunk driving is taken for granted among bar drinkers. An observational study of drinkers in a variety of southern California bars noted, "[D]rinking-driving is the normal, expected behavior of bar patrons. It is the absence of it, the failure to drive after drinking, that bar patrons must account for to each other" (Gusfield, Rasmussen, and Kotarba, 1984: 47).

The prevalence of serving practices leading to highly impairing BACs was explored in an informal study in which staff members of a safety organization were sent to various bars in a small Ohio city (Highway Safety Foundation, 1972). They were instructed to order "with the objective of determining how many drinks he could obtain before his service would be terminated by the bartender." Despite unanimous agreement by local bartenders in a prior survey that they should limit service to prevent excessive drinking, the foundation's staff achieved impressive consumption without ever being cut off. The results of five bar visits were as follows: one person was able to order fifteen drinks in slightly more than 2 hours (with an additional five being served in other premises later on that day); a second consumed seven drinks in 1½ hours; a third was served six double drinks in less than 2 hours; a fourth bought eleven beers in less than two hours; and a fifth person was served fourteen drinks in about 1½ hours. Three of the five staffers attained BACs in excess of 0.20 percent. Notes taken by observers testified that all these individuals exhibited clear signs of impairment. The study concluded that bartenders at all sites were aware of the subjects' impaired condition, and that they were both ignorant about potential abuse of alcohol and "not concerned with problem consumption."

Heavy drinking in bars is produced by the coincidence of economic incentives for management with social incentives provided by patrons. Again, as stated by Gusfield, Rasmussen, and Kotarba (1984: 51): "A fundamental fact about the bar in American life is that it is a business. It operates in a market economy in which budgets, expenses, profits and losses are essential considerations. Bar owners are in the business of buying and selling liquor." This fact leads to a variety of practices meant to stimulate sales and increase alcohol consumption. Examples are promotions and discounts at slow times (happy hours), basing sales on credit rather than cash (running a tab), and suggesting reorders (hustling drinks). These practices resonate with certain clients' customs, such as the buying of rounds among friends and competitive consumption games, to produce an environment conducive to consuming large quantities of alcohol.

Moreover, there are norms in the bar environment that discourage being concerned with drunk driving and intervening to prevent it. The "beer culture" (Berger and Snortum, 1985), with its norms encouraging heavy consumption, is centered in certain kinds of bars. In these same bars, norms may also discourage intervention to prevent impaired patrons from driving. To imply that someone may have drunk too much to drive safely impugns his competency as a drinker and thus his social standing. Expressing concern for someone, especially a stranger, may violate standards of privacy, while marking the one concerned as being timid or prudish.

As Gusfield, Rasmussen, and Kotarba (1984) note, servers often experience difficulties in perceiving and responding to the danger of drunk driving by the clientele. In many kinds of bars and taverns, crowd size and impersonality interfere with management's ability to know how much is being consumed, and the difficulty of identifying alcohol impairment confounds reliable identification of those needing control. Furthermore, although bar managements are aware of and concerned about the possibilities of "trouble" as a consequence of drinking, consequences outside the premises are not usually taken into account. The researchers summarized bar management's perceptions as follows:

Trouble is something that can happen inside the bar and not outside. Things outside the bar, regardless of whether they originated in the bar, are not troublesome.

Drinking-driving is not trouble for bars or bartenders. It does not disrupt the setting. The bar's economic interest is not affected. No legal prohibition is violated by the bar when its patron is arrested for drinking-driving or involved in an accident. Police do not enter the premises. [55]

Service practices The hope that bar managements might be effective as allies in reducing drunk driving has led to the formation of programs for training alcohol servers. Popular programs offering relatively intensive training include the Training for Intervention Procedures by Servers of Alcohol (TIPS) and Training in Alcohol Management (TAM) programs sponsored by the major brewing companies. The objectives of these programs include imparting knowledge of techniques for keeping patrons from reaching high BACs, especially those that are illegal when driving; not serving underaged patrons or those "over the limit"; and providing safe rides home for patrons requiring them. Among the techniques taught for controlling consumption by problematic customers are offering food or nonalcoholic drinks, delaying service, reducing the alcoholic content of drinks served, and, ultimately, refusing service.

Pilot studies of server training have reported optimistic findings (e.g., Saltz, 1987; Russ and Geller, 1987). Trained servers have increased their relevant knowledge. They use intervention techniques more than they did before training and more than untrained personnel in matched facilities. However, establishments participating in the pilot studies are not a representative sample of bars. Their willingness to participate in training and evaluation research probably indicates that their managements are more conscientious than those in most retail establishments. Moreover, all the evaluations have been short-term, providing no basis on which to predict the durability of changes in server behavior. Most important, even though training produced changes, large proportions of apparently impaired and even illegal drivers were still being served, and the ultimate sanction of cutting off the drinker was very rarely used by the trained servers.

The largest-scale evaluation of server training to date (McKnight, 1988) employed observers feigning intoxication while demanding service. In sites in eight states a model training program was administered to volunteers from 100 alcohol-selling establishments, which were paired with 138 control establishments. The "intoxicated" pseudo-patrons succeeded in being served without any intervention about 86 percent of the time prior to staff training, but only about 73 percent of the time after training, in the cooperating establishments. They were served about 83 percent of the time in the control establishments.

Although this general result can be viewed as encouraging, testifying to increases in servers' awareness of and motivation to do something about intoxication, there were no interventions of any kind in nearly three-quarters of the observations in premises with trained servers. In addition, the bulk of interventions that did occur were only partial, such as asking about the patron's condition. Full interventions, involving refusal to serve the "intoxicated" persons, increased merely from about 5 percent prior to training to about 7 percent after. In the matter of this central goal, namely, increasing compliance to the law prohibiting serving intoxicated people, the results are disappointing. Furthermore, in three of the eight states there were no significant increases in server interventions following training. This fact could not be explained as a reflection of different liability laws.

Observers attempting to purchase impairing quantities of drinks were also used in a study of Utah's mandatory training program (Howard-Pitney et al., 1991). In this study, both servers and managers received training. The study compared behavior of personnel in thirteen establishments experiencing the training programs with those in eleven matched control establishments. No significant differences were observed in the numbers of interventions, which were rare in both groups of establishments.

The limitations of server training appear to be due in part to the lack of incentives to take production of drunk drivers into account in the management of the bar business. No amount of server training is likely to produce important behavior changes without the support of management policies. Among the functions required of management are providing and requiring the necessary training; upholding decisions by service personnel to intervene in specific cases and compensating for income (tips) lost owing to compliance with training principles; and sanctioning laxness in complying with the rules.

In most markets, bar management experiences little incentive to fulfill these functions. Other things being equal, the more drinks sold, the greater the rewards to both servers and managers. Indeed, were server intervention both aggressive and successful, the economic health of many drinking establishments might be threatened. Robert Hammond, director of the Alcohol Research Information Service, has stated that if all drinkers were to consume no more than what is regarded as the maximum "moderate" amount of alcohol—an average of about two drinks per day—the alcoholic beverage industry would experience "a whopping 40 percent decrease in the sale of beer, wine and distilled spirits, based on 1981 sales figures" (cited in Langton, 1991: 147–48). Based on the previously cited case studies of patrons exiting bars, it appears that many bars would have to cut off service to the majority of their customers in order to keep their BACs below 0.10 percent on departure.

What is more, the damage produced by the drunk drivers is literally externalized—removed from management calculations and decisions—in the absence of effective liability laws or equivalent regulations. In such circumstances, to garner support for server intervention among bar managers may require not only acknowledgment of the linkage between what happens in the bar and what happens on the road, but also the prodding of conscience against the imperatives of economics. A certain segment of the bar trade, one that produces considerable numbers of drunk drivers, can be expected to ignore the linkage and to reject any appeals of conscience. For such establishments in particular, it is unreasonable to expect much improvement from server training without further motivating conditions.

A change in the legal environment might provide a background for more significant accomplishments from server training. This approach has been promoted by James Mosher and his associates in the Model Alcoholic Beverage Retail Licensee Liability Act of 1985 (e.g., Colman, Well, and Mosher, 1985; Saltz, 1989). This proposed law would establish civil liability for both negligent and reckless service of alcoholic beverages, but would allow establishments to plead adherence to "responsible business practices" as a defense. These practices include server training and effective management policies supporting application of the training. Inasmuch as exposure to the risk of lawsuits posed by this legislation would still be a matter of small probabilities that could be disregarded by cynical or hopeful managements, incorporation of the defense advantages into insurance premiums might be expected to accelerate the adoption of the responsible practices. Indeed, some insurance companies currently offer discounts on liquor law liability coverage to bars that train sufficient numbers of their servers in recognized programs.

The model act has been adopted by a few states and is now being considered by others. Additional laws regulating the on-premise sale of liquor—including prohibitions on serving underaged and intoxicated persons that are typically enforced by liquor control authorities—may also stimulate interest in and support for server intervention. Whether important and lasting changes in server behavior can be achieved should be determinable in the near future. There are serious constraints on what can be expected from these laws, in the form of short-run economic advantages—for the establishment as a whole and for individual servers—in selling alcohol to customers likely to drive. Such customers purchase large quantities of the bar's stock in trade and probably account for large proportions of the establishment's profit and the server's tips. Additional problems lie in the difficulty of reliably detecting alcohol impairment at BACs likely to produce considerable risk and in the application of interventions in skillful ways so as not to discourage repeat business. Policy makers concerned with reducing drunk driving can hardly oppose instituting server training and providing the necessary legal and financial bases for its use. However, expectations of benefits ought, in my opinion, to be modest.

Other service policies and customs Certain alcoholic beverage marketing practices, unobjectionable when applied to many consumer products, appear to have the undesirable effect of increasing the alcohol consumption of drivers to risky levels. Discounts and promotions, notably the happy hour, which often coincides with commuting time, have been principally at issue. Babor and his colleagues, in both experimental and field studies, confirm that reduced-price promotions can be enormously successful in increasing alcohol sales and consumption. Moreover, the happy hour is found to have its intended effect of initiating drinking episodes that continue once prices return to regular levels. Babor's experimental findings are indeed startling: "When the purchase price was reduced by half, casual and heavy drinkers increased their consumption eight and nine times, respectively, over that of comparable subjects without happy hour" (Babor et al., 1978: 39). In a field study at a small-town tavern, "Nonhappy-hour patrons drank an average of 3.73 drinks per day and happy-hour patrons 9.56" (Babor et al., 1980: 643). Methodological questions about the size and representativeness of the samples in these studies can be raised, and at least one observational study (Smart and Adlaf, 1986) has failed to find predicted reductions in drinking as a consequence of a ban on happy hours. However, Babor's studies confirm expectations based on intuition, common sense, and economic theory: if the price goes down, consumption goes up. It seems reasonable to recommend at least provisionally that restrictions on price promotions be enacted into codes regulating the sale of liquor in bars and taverns. Such restrictions would also apply to single-price, or "drink-and-drown," promotions, which may lead to intoxication in the way that buffet dinners lead to indigestion. Restrictions should also apply to free drinks, which Gusfield, Rasmussen, and Kotarba (1984) found were frequently offered at bar closing times; they noted that these were often the strongest drinks of the evening, served just before the customers drove home.

Certain other marketing practices associated with heavy drinking in bars might also be restricted. For instance, Geller, Russ, and Altomari (1986) found that drinkers ordering beer by the pitcher consumed an average of thirty-nine ounces per sitting, whereas those ordering by the bottle or glass consumed an average of twelve to fifteen ounces per sitting. Although some of this excess no doubt reflects the heavy drinker's anticipation and desire to save money by ordering in quantity, part of it may be due to the stimulation of consumption by the abundance provided. It appears reasonable to require that drinks be served in individual servings containing no more than a standard, for example, one-half ounce, dose of pure alcohol. Regulations should be devised for the purpose of reducing the practice of hustling drinks. For instance, servers could be prohibited from suggesting drink orders or refills.

Some current business practices that research suggests *diminish* the likelihood of drunk driving should be encouraged through legal mandates. Providing food, which tends to lower peak BACs, can be encouraged by adopting regulations that require bars to show a certain proportion of food sales or to keep snacks on hand. Designated driver arrangements, if found in further research to yield net health benefits, can be encouraged, for instance, by requiring servers to ask parties arriving together whether there is a nondrinking driver for the group. Requiring licensed premises to remain open for at least an hour beyond the time for serving alcoholic beverages, during which food and nonalcoholic beverages could be sold, is another possibility. This staged closing might prevent the bunching of impaired drivers on the road at closing time and permit some amount of alcohol to be metabolized before driving.

There are also opportunities to influence alcohol service in private premises. Private parties contribute a relatively small proportion of the drunk drivers on the road, but this source should not be totally neglected. In conjunction with media promotion of slogans like "Friends don't let friends drive drunk," hosts should be taught to recognize the signs of intoxication (McKnight and Marques, 1990). It might also be possible to suggest specific measures that hosts could use to help ensure their guests' safety. Examples include advice to refrain from serving carbonated mixers, which tend to accelerate absorption of alcohol; to refrain from refilling glasses except on request; to replace alcohol service with coffee service before guests start to depart; and to be alert to people who might benefit from riding home with others and to those who might safely be trusted with providing such transportation (American Automobile Association, 1990). Taking a cue from Norwegian practice, hosts could be advised to offer overnight hospitality to guests who consume a great deal of alcohol. It has been suggested that hosts would pay more attention to advice like this if they were financially liable for damage produced by their guests while driving home. However, this suggestion does not rest on scientific evidence, and one may have doubts about the possibility of communicating liability rules to noncommercial servers of alcohol so as to change their behavior.

Many of the ideas in this section are not based on research and are offered as reasonable but unproven suggestions that might offer a modicum of control over BACs reached by drinkers. They are symbolically appropriate in all events. However, it is unrealistic to expect major saving of lives from controls that fail to challenge the status of alcoholic beverages as a conventional market commodity. Having that status, alcohol may be distributed in ways that do not distinguish it from other legal goods. In particular, there are few laws to prevent its being promoted and sold with the sole goal of maximizing profit. Major success in the effort to save lives now lost to drunk driving and other alcohol-related problems probably requires rejection or at least modification of this status.

Marketing constraints

As legal products, thus far regarded as being minimally different from other goods on the market, alcoholic beverages are aggressively promoted in the United States. Brewers in particular devote enormous resources to sponsorships and promotions of their product. The principal means of marketing, and the one that has had the most critical examination, is advertising.

Expenditures on advertising of alcoholic beverages amount to well over $1 billion per year (Cowan and Mosher, 1985: 637) and, as noted previously, amount to substantial fractions of the budgets of the major media in this country. Most of these messages feature "attractive and youthful (but not underage) characters display[ing] enjoyment (but not intoxication). Among the benefits frequently linked to alcohol are social camaraderie, romance, masculinity/femininity, adventure, relaxation, and elegance" (Atkin, 1989: 18). Beer, which is especially marketed to men, "is represented as the medium through which one demonstrates one's masculinity, is initiated into the adult world, communicates with other men, expresses feelings towards them, preserves and recaptures the history of one's group of male friends, and makes romantic contacts with women" (Postman et al., 1987: 48).

The rationale given by brewing executives for these expenses is to increase the market for the brands being advertised, but not to increase the overall consumption of beer. This claim is a standard response to critics of advertising who maintain that it persuades people to buy things they do not need or should not have (Schudson, 1984: 9), and it is stated seriously by beer advertisers. In the words of congressional testimony by representatives of a major brewer, "The purpose *and effect* of beer advertising is to create brand loyalty—not to increase the total amount of beer consumed in our society. Beer advertising has *no significant impact* on overall consumption, and *does not* cause abusive drinking or drinking among underage individuals" (cited in Ross, 1986: 501). Furthermore, representatives of the industry vehemently assert their watchfulness against suggesting the appropriateness of drinking and driving. Content analysis of advertisements confirms that vehicles are seldom depicted, and drinking with driving is never shown (Atkin, 1989: 19).

The effects of alcohol advertising The fact that alcohol producers admit the potential of advertising to increase consumption of advertised brands and back up this admission by making an enormous investment in the enterprise is hard to reconcile with their denial that total consumption of alcoholic beverages can be increased at the expense of other beverages. As Cowan and Mosher (1985) convincingly argue, the idea of an overall beverage market that includes both alcoholic and nonalcoholic drinks makes sense to business. Within this market, substitutions occur. Citing the publication *Beverage Industry*, Cowan and Mosher note that soft drinks, tap water, coffee, beer, and milk—in that order, each with at least a 10 percent segment—are the principal components of this market. Shifts in the relative shares of the beverage market take place over time, while the total consumption per capita remains about the same. In recent years, the share going to coffee and milk has declined, that going to beer has increased modestly, and that of soft drinks has increased impressively. The major loser has been tap water. A not unreasonable hypothesis is that advertising expenditures have been partly responsible for this shift in which highly advertised commercial beverages have grown at the expense of the less advertised, and advertised beverages have prospered at the expense of the unadvertised one—the virtually free tap water.

Contrary to expectations, the scientific literature has not provided strong support for this hypothesis. Relevant studies include laboratory experiments, econometric analyses of the relationship between advertising expenses and alcohol consumption and problems, and statistical analyses of the relationship between these measures and exposure to advertising. The reviews of this literature differ in their conclusions. On the one hand, for example, Atkin, Neuendorf, and McDermott (1983: 323) conclude, "The correlational findings show that alcohol advertising exposure is positively related to heavy drinking, problem drinking, and hazardous drinking. The relationships are moderate in strength for the heavy drinking and drinking/driving indices." On the other hand, Smart (1988: 321) concludes, "Current research suggests that advertising is, at best, a weak variable affecting alcohol consumption. It would be better if those interested in effective alcohol controls spent time controlling prices and availability rather than controlling advertising."

The ambiguous research findings may indicate that, in the complicated world of social causation, the effect of advertising is not sufficiently great to be distinguished from that of other factors that influence alcohol consumption and problems, including other marketing tools

(Schudson, 1984). In addition, the research in question is essentially limited to identifying short-term effects, but it is likely that advertising's effects may be greater in the long run, where effectiveness is far more difficult to demonstrate, than in the short run. As Holder (1987) notes,

Researchers have a difficult, if not impossible, task to demonstrate that alcohol advertising unilaterally causes alcohol problems. Advertisements are but a part of all mass messages. Their effect is cumulative. . . . Alcohol advertising and drinking are part of a complex, nonlinear system with multiple levels of feedback and lagged response. . . . Linear statistics, the techniques most frequently used by behavioral scientists, has limited applicability in such situations.

This interpretation is supported by research concerned not with consumption or problems, but with the formation of attitudes about alcoholic beverages. Wallack, Cassady and Grube (1990) studied the effects of televised beer commercials on fifth- and sixth-grade children. They found that most of the children, especially the boys, were frequently exposed to such commercials (generally through sports programming). This exposure was related to such matters as belief in the truth of the messages, positive beliefs about the use of beer, and expectations of drinking as an adult.

In brief, social science research has not given unambiguous support to the hypothesis that exposure to alcohol advertising increases consumption—but it is not well suited to providing such support. From the viewpoint of reducing drunk driving, the hypothesized relationship is not unreasonable as grounds on which to base social policy. However, if policies in this category are adopted, the lack of a strong knowledge base should be recognized; commitment to them should be provisional, and implementation should be done with an eye to maximizing opportunities for evaluation.

Possibilities for restricting advertising The messages contained in alcohol advertising are objectionable to the extent they imply that any amount of drinking in conjunction with driving is compatible with traffic safety. Direct encouragement of this behavior would be unconscionable. It is not a matter of actual concern, since there are few alcohol advertisements today in which cars are even depicted (though beer company sponsorship of motor sports is common and certainly raises questions of propriety—see Buchanan and Lev, 1990).

However, mere depiction of drinking in settings that are normally reached by car, such as in taverns or out-of-doors, may be regarded as an inappropriate message from the viewpoint of avoiding drunk driving. Messages like "Know your limits" and "Know when to say when" seem to suggest that a moderate BAC might be tolerable for normal, routine, activities, including driving, and such a suggestion is clearly misleading. Indeed, promotion of the positive aspects of consumption with no mention of the dangers seems most inappropriate when dealing with a drug that has dangerous ˙de effects. In the words of Mosher and Wallack (1989: 103), "Alcoholic beverage advertising is misleading in two ways: (1) Alcoholic beverages are promoted by appeals to desires and needs that are irrelevant to the product; and, (2) The absence of accurate health information in the marketing of a product with serious public health consequences hampers the consumer in making an informed choice."

If one accepts the view that alcohol is, among other things, a potentially dangerous drug, a case can be made that it should not be advertised at all. Even highly beneficent and legal medicinal drugs may be promoted only to specialists, such as physicians, and this model can be adopted in order to reduce the dissemination of misleading messages that accompany much current alcohol advertising. Although direct evidence on the effect of alcohol advertising prohibitions may be thin, there is now considerable evidence from bans and controls on tobacco advertising that such policies can reduce consumption, especially among young people (Toxic Substances Board, 1989a; 1989b; Warner, 1989). This offers a basis for hopes of achieving similar results for alcohol.

In spite of the possible benefits of this approach, even such staunch critics of alcoholic beverage advertising as Atkin (1989: 28) have, because of the relatively modest effects demonstrated in research and pragmatic political considerations, stopped short of recommending broad-scale restrictions. It may be more realistic to demand that both the industry and regulatory agencies scrutinize the claims made in alcohol advertising more carefully and that advertising in favor of liquor consumption be balanced by public health advertising emphasizing its dangers. To quote Holder (1987) once more, "Perhaps, the most significant issue for alcohol abuse prevention is the normalization of alcohol through advertising and beverage promotion. Normalization does not inform us about the consequences of high-risk consumption.

114

It can create a misleading impression that drinking is always harmless." Counteradvertising to neutralize this message was recently proposed by the prestigious, bipartisan National Commission on Drug-Free Schools (1990). The commission projected funding the campaign through a tax on alcohol and tobacco advertising. In a current example of counteradvertising for smoking, for example, a physicians' group, Doctors Ought to Care (DOC), has been distributing material entitled "The Camel's Lumps" that depicts a well-known cigarette's mascot as the victim of disfiguring cancer. Perhaps the image of Spuds McKenzie on a stretcher in a hospital emergency room might make the point for his sponsor's product. Messages opposed to those conveyed in alcohol advertising might also have an appropriate place in school health curricula.

Finally, whether or not restrictions are considered, the public subsidy of alcohol advertising through tax breaks to liquor producers, who are permitted to deduct the cost of advertising from their taxable income, seems inappropriate. Withdrawal of that subsidy neither raises the issues of free speech attending limitations and bans nor involves the costs of producing and distributing counteradvertising. Assuming that the courts find the measure constitutionally permissible, ending the tax deductibility of advertising for alcohol and other recreational drugs seems a reasonable, appropriate, and feasible element in the effort to reduce drunk driving.

Countermeasures based in alcohol policy are premised on the understanding that driving is nearly universal in American society, and therefore that much of the drinking that takes place is likely to be associated with driving. Given that BACs produced by even socially acceptable drinking are associated with significant increases in the risk of fatal crashes, reduction of drinking in general can be seen as a useful lifesaving measure. Policies that are effective in reducing heavy drinking or those kinds of drinking most likely to be accompanied by driving should be especially effective in saving lives, but general drinking reductions can also be expected to produce important reductions in drunk driving.

Among the countermeasures based in alcohol policy, research supports the expectation that intervening in the market through taxation is likely to be effective. Although one can argue with the precise estimates offered in the relevant studies, there is little scholarly disagreement with the prediction that increased prices reduce consumption of alcoholic beverages and that reduced consumption results in the diminution of alcohol-related problems, including drunk driving.

Taxation has several features to recommend it, beyond its likely effectiveness. It is popular in principle with the public and is difficult to evade. By forcing the price of the product to cover social costs currently externalized, it is economically rational. It is also ethical, in that it respects the freedom of the individual to make an unwise choice, provided the social costs of that choice are paid.

Other forms of market control offer additional opportunities for reducing alcohol consumption and problems, though in more complicated and less reliable ways. On the whole, they offer small improvements that may justify their cost. They cannot, however, be expected to have major effects, comparable to those expected of taxation. Indeed, some existing market interventions, such as extensive controls on times and location of alcohol sales, appear to produce few results and might be abandoned.

Server intervention stands out as directed precisely at reducing the most dangerous alcohol consumption, drinking to intoxication at locations where the drinker is likely to drive. Moreover, training programs offer possibilities of cooperation with the hospitality industry. However, the economic and legal decks are stacked against maximum use of what can be taught in these programs. Unless the underlying liabilities and regulations are adjusted, for example by "dram shop" laws, so that drunk driving becomes "trouble" for the personnel and management of bars and taverns, server training is likely to be of marginal importance in reducing drunk driving.

No reasonable, effective, and efficient drunk driving countermeasure should be omitted from public policy merely because its contribution is small relative to the yield from other policies. All such measures should be included in the total package of policies, to the extent that resources permit. Control of drunk driving will never be complete, but we are in a position to reduce the current toll importantly, by adopting a policy package in which alcohol-based countermeasures play a central role.

Countermeasures Based in Transportation Policy

Countermeasures that use transportation policy are premised on the assumption that drunk driving can be reduced by reducing miles traveled by private automobiles. This premise parallels the one underlying countermeasures based in alcohol policy, that is, that drunk driving can be reduced by reducing alcohol consumption. Both types of measures are founded on the understanding that drunk driving is caused by accepted institutional arrangements. If the problem lies in the conjunction of two institutions, then changing either one can reduce the problem by reducing the intersection even though the other institution is unchanged. Of course, if both drinking and driving were reduced, greater reductions in drunk driving could be expected, other things being equal, and if driving reductions were concentrated on occasions associated with drinking, their effect would be greater yet. Furthermore, reduced automobile mileage achieved through concern with drunk driving will affect other social problems. One may count as benefits from policies related to reducing the amount of driving in society any reductions coincidentally produced in such problems as highway congestion and air pollution.

Countermeasures based in transportation policy have played a much smaller role in the policy discussion surrounding drunk driving than have those based in alcohol policy. One reason is that reductions in automobile use are difficult to achieve. While the word *addiction* is less often heard in discussing driving than in discussing drinking, driving's highly inelastic relationship with cost and inconvenience is even more firmly

5

established. If it is hard to conceive of an alcoholic reducing his drug intake, it is even more difficult to conceive of an American motorist reducing his mileage. Yet evidence indicates that these reductions are possible. Even within recent memory, American driving patterns and mileage were reduced as a result of an oil crisis, and numerous lives were saved as a result.

In 1974, tensions in the Middle East caused supplies of oil from the Persian Gulf to be interrupted. Among the consequences for Americans was a gasoline shortage, higher gas prices, long lines for fuel, and reduced hours of operation for gas stations. It became risky to travel long distances, given the uncertainty of refueling. That year vehicle mileage in the United States declined for the first time since 1946— by 1.45 percent. If the mileage-based fatality rate for 1974 had been the same as for 1973, eight hundred more deaths would have resulted. (The actual saving, projecting a long-term decline in that rate, was probably somewhat less.)

The gas crisis is not raised to suggest model policy. Driving reduction taken to an extreme would eliminate crash fatalities altogether by eliminating automotive transportation—a clearly unrealistic proposition. Rather, the example is cited to establish the principle that if automobile mileage is lowered to some extent, some lives will be saved. How society should reduce mileage is a political judgment, just as it is with alcohol consumption. In this judgment, both the costs and benefits associated with the reduced consumption or mileage must be considered.

One of the most effective means of reducing the use of automobiles would be to significantly increase the price of fuel. Increasing the gasoline tax is one means of accomplishing this. The idea of taxing fuel in order to reduce drunk driving is not commonly interjected into today's deterrence-dominated discourse, but it has been proposed for this purpose by public health professionals (Beauchamp, 1983). Reductions in automobile use occasioned by more expensive fuel would most likely be concentrated in "discretionary," or recreational, driving, precisely the kind most likely to be alcohol-impaired. Thus, expected reductions in drunk driving should exceed the overall change in miles traveled. Although large fuel tax increases in the United States are unlikely to be enacted solely on the basis of reducing drunk driving, this benefit should be presented alongside considerations of environmental quality, defense, deficit reduction, and other benefits in supporting proposals for higher taxes. Increases in the normal price of fuel in recent years, partly due to modestly higher federal and state taxes, may well reduce future travel. Although the rising cost of energy creates an economic cloud for many, it may have a silver lining in the form of saved lives.

In contrast to the case of alcohol-tax increases for the purpose of reducing drinking, the American public resents fuel tax increases. Raising fuel taxes to reduce driving will thus not easily be embraced in the foreseeable future. However, other kinds of countermeasures based in transportation policy can be offered with the expectation that they will gain political support. Being directed at the institutional causes of drunk driving, they form an important part of society's potential arsenal of countermeasures for this social problem. The following discussion treats them as either providing alternatives or reducing access to driving.

Providing alternatives to driving

Alternatives to driving are hard to envisage because the automobile has become such an essential element of almost every community and neighborhood it has touched. In the words of a prestigious group of international experts formed to consider the future of traffic safety,

> Foremost in consideration of [reducing mileage] must be the realisation that extensive reliance on exposure control sets up major conflicts with other values important in many societies, touching on such basic issues as the ready ability to choose where to work and live, the very layout of cities, and the freedom of movement considered a keystone of the political system in many countries. [Trinca et al., 1988: 65]

The physical structure of the United States is conditioned on the assumption that all adults can drive. Thus, urban residential density is low, as large numbers of people fulfill the dream of our English forefathers to live in a castle in a park. This ideal prevails even though the castle be a mobile home and the park the size of a postage stamp. Unlike many Europeans, Americans with means generally prefer to live at the periphery of the metropolitan area, not in its center, and certainly not in multistory buildings or row houses. Likewise, the traditional pattern of employment and recreation being located downtown has been largely replaced with suburbanized shopping malls and office

119

parks. Mass transit, designed to serve the centralized urban center, in the twentieth century has first become noncompetitive and then irrelevant to the physical layout of the metropolitan community. For most people living in this community, all activities, with the exception of neighborly sociability and elementary schooling, are premised on use of the automobile. In short, driving has become a necessity (Schneider, 1971).

Planning for urban density

An unregulated real estate market can probably be expected to continue the centrifugal, low-density pattern observable in all recently developed American cities. Driving will continue to be a necessity for all purposes, including recreation and drinking. This development pattern, I maintain, sets the stage for drunk driving as a social problem.

Intervening in the market in order to encourage denser residential patterns and more extensive local services should produce less driving in general and less impaired driving. There is empirical evidence consistent with this proposition from densely populated American cities. New York City appears to have a very low rate of drunk driving. While it contains roughly 40 percent of the state's population, the city has historically generated only about 3 percent of the state's drunk-driving convictions. Although this fact can be interpreted in other ways, the impression of minimal involvement by New Yorkers in drunk driving is supported in surveys. A study of New York high school students found 11 percent of those in the city admitting drunk (or drugged) driving in the previous year, compared with 28 percent in the suburbs and 29 percent upstate (Barnes and Welte, 1988a). Another New York survey of adults eighteen years of age and older (Barnes and Welte, 1988b) obtained similar findings and presented a more detailed explanation:

> The rate of driving under the effects of alcohol is twice as great in both suburban New York City (16%) and Upstate areas (19%) as in New York City (8%). . . . The regional variations in the rates of driving are also vastly different, with 44% of New York City residents indicating that they do not drive and 10% and 14%, respectively, of suburban New Yorkers and Upstate New Yorkers indicating that they do not drive. However, if the rates of driving under the effects of alcohol were recalculated based on *drivers only*,

Upstate New York still has a greater proportion of adults reporting driving under alcohol's effects (22%) than New York City (14%) with the proportion in New York City suburbs being between the other two areas. [63]

Surveys of young people in a variety of other American communities found that in Washington, D.C., youths are far less likely to report drunk driving (lifetime incidence of 15.1 percent) than they are in, for example, Los Angeles (39.2 percent), Omaha (58.5 percent), or the small town of Espanola, New Mexico (59.9 percent) (Klitzner, Vegega, and Gruenewald, 1988). The denser layout of places like New York and Washington renders driving less necessary and less convenient, while drinking establishments are more likely to be reachable without the use of a car.

The suggestion that urban density be increased and that facilities be located closer to residences in order to counter the centrifugal effects of a century of the automobile on land development must be regarded as applicable mainly in the long run. Although increased urban density in America may be thought of as essential and even inevitable because of the waste of limited resources implicit in current residential patterns, the notion conflicts with cultural standards of housing. Most Americans probably find the life-style of Lake Shore Drive or Third Avenue less appealing than that of Lake Forest or Great Neck. However, moderately dense housing has proved attractive in numerous urban enclaves inhabited by people with ample alternative housing possibilities: I refer to such places as Beacon Hill in Boston, Washington's Georgetown, and San Francisco's Pacific Heights. These are neighborhoods of great amenity and prestige, but also areas in which the use of cars, especially for recreational purposes, is inconvenient and frequently unnecessary. A more general endorsement of the virtues of this life-style is available in Jane Jacobs's classic *Death and Life of Great American Cities* (1963), among other works. It seems reasonable to think that encouragement of similar residential textures through zoning and tax incentives could produce a reduction in automobile usage.

Specific regulations could address the siting of bars and taverns with reference to both neighborhoods and highways. It would be possible to discourage on-premise sales outlets for alcohol in locations that can be reached easily by no means other than driving, for example, in shopping malls and roadside strips as opposed to neighborhood centers.

Such developments could be discouraged through zoning regulations and tax incentives (Wittman, 1986).

It is not necessary to await massive urban renewal or the construction of entirely new towns and cities to use planning tools to reduce drunk driving. Reasonable speculation, based on a modest amount of data, suggests the usefulness of zoning and other regulatory policies for discouraging driving that may be linked with drinking. The expected outcome of short-term planning interventions is unlikely to be spectacular, but the task of reducing drunk driving is of sufficient importance that we should welcome minor as well as major contributions. Long-term planning may make a larger difference in the cities of the future.

Subsidized alternative transportation

Rather than increasing the cost of automobile use, transportation-based policy can focus on providing attractive alternatives for leisure occasions when drinking is likely. A model for this approach is the program devised by Notre Dame University at a time when Indiana's drinking age was higher than that in nearby Michigan. The university administration recognized that large numbers of students were driving from the campus across the state line in order to drink in Michigan bars, and this was resulting in much impaired driving and consequent injuries and deaths. The problem was relieved by providing university buses to transport drinkers to and from the state line (Gusfield, 1982).

A general version of this countermeasure, suitable mainly for large and densely built cities, would be to encourage the use of mass transit for recreational travel. Drinking trips that rely on the use of mass transit do not produce drunk driving. However, to be used, transit must be available, in time as well as in place. In Washington, D.C., for example, the subway trains stop running at midnight, long before the bars close, and this discourages drinkers from traveling by train to drinking locations. Such disjunctions of transit hours and drinking hours could be remedied by lengthening the period of service.

However, under most circumstances in America, the car has almost insurmountable advantages over mass transit in cost and convenience. Subways and buses in this country are often viewed as being unreliable, slow, dirty, dangerous, and expensive. Unfortunately, expense is among the least of mass transit's problems, and even extensive fare subsidies may not be able to increase ridership to an important degree at most times in most places.

The only mode of public transportation in general use today with a reasonable chance of being competitive with the private automobile as a conveyance to and from drinking activities is the taxicab. In terms of speed and flexibility of routing it is the equal of the car. Although many units fall short in terms of comfort, this disadvantage is remediable; the taxi's main inherent shortcoming is cost. If one overlooks the fixed costs of car ownership, such as depreciation and insurance, and counts only the variable ones like gasoline and parking fees, taxis are typically much more expensive than private automobiles. There may be additional reasons for preferring the car, including immediate availability, privacy, and the opportunity to display taste or wealth; but if the cost barrier were lowered, it is possible that many people could be lured from their cars when traveling to and from drinking activities. Taxi use would be relatively more attractive when parking at the destination is congested and expensive and when police patrols present realistic threats to drunk drivers.

It would be most effective for reducing drunk driving if people both arrived at and departed from drinking occasions by cab. This feature is missing from the safe rides programs discussed below. People driving their cars on drinking occasions are discouraged from using alternative transportation once they have consumed alcohol by the need to retrieve the cars. The simplest way of encouraging round-trip use of alternative transportation would be to subsidize it. Inasmuch as a subsidy specific to drinking destinations would be cumbersome and probably unworkable, the subsidy would most simply cover all travel during recreational or drinking hours. If some people used the cheaper cabs for going to Mass instead of to the bar, this use and subsidy would be justified on the grounds that it is necessary in order to subsidize the drinking trip and perhaps also that it is better to leave driving at these more hazardous hours to professionals in all cases.

Subsidized taxicab programs would be more feasible in some communities than in others. Very small towns (under ten thousand people) may be unable to support cab service at any price, while in some large cities, where routine trips are likely to involve long distances, keeping costs within reason may make it difficult to offer attractively priced service. However, subsidizing of taxis does not seem to be prima facie impractical in middle-sized cities with existing taxi fleets and moderate distances within their borders.

Subsidized alternative transportation may not be cheap, but its costs are not likely to be considered unbearable if it achieves substantial reductions in drunk driving. In 1990, the average cab ride in the forty largest American cities was 4.7 miles (International Taxicab Association, 1990). Trips from downtown points to airports of as much as 20 to 25 miles were an important fraction of the total, so that this figure probably overestimates the mileage involved in drinking trips. At average cab rates prevailing in 1990, the 4.7-mile trip would have cost $7.41, but there were considerable price differences among cities, a function of the different local markets. At rates prevailing in Tulsa, Oklahoma, for example, the 4.7-mile trip would have cost $5.75.

According to Edward G. Davis, research director of the International Taxicab Association, additional nighttime business would be eagerly sought by cab companies, as they typically have no more than a quarter to a third of their fleet on the roads at midnight. They would be likely to view such a service as good public relations and as a way to stimulate demand for their services at other times of day. A request for bids to provide general nighttime service might yield very attractive rates per trip. Thus, especially if a token charge, for example, the equivalent of a rush-hour bus fare, were paid by riders, the subsidy required would probably be manageable in many cities.

This issue has been the topic of some informal discussions at meetings on safety policy, but these have not led to policy interventions, even on an experimental basis. Joseph Gusfield frequently begins his lectures on dealing with drunk driving by asking that representatives of the taxi industry in the audience raise their hands. Typically, none are present, making the point that even interests standing to profit from such a policy have failed to see it as a live issue. It has been invisible from other perspectives as well. Representatives of a large brewing company once asked me how they could spend a large sum of money on a demonstration project for reducing drunk driving. My suggestion of subsidizing nighttime cab service in a medium-sized city was rejected on the ground that it did not deal with drunk driving. As a consequence of these perceptions, there is little experience, much less evaluation, relevant to the topic. Some public transit systems, including those in Toronto, New York, Boston, and Milwaukee, have in the past offered free bus and subway carriage on holidays like New Year's Eve, and in interviews with the press officials have claimed reduced impaired driving; but these interventions are far more limited than a general program of subsidized taxi fares would be, and none has been subjected to competent evaluation.

The size of the subsidy required will depend largely on the success of the program. As noted below, current safe rides programs, which offer impaired drivers free rides home, have proved to be quite economical, but they have been relatively little used. The more successful the taxi subsidy program—that is, the more it is used and the fewer the limitations on the areas and distances served—the more costly it would be. The cash price of a trip would have to be set in light of both the degree of inducement to use the system and the amount of resources available for its support. The source of funds would condition the latter. (One potentially lucrative source might be a surtax on drinks served in bars, which would both support the alternative transportation program and reduce consumption of drinks by those who nonetheless chose to drive.) The subsidy program is envisaged as furnishing trips during all usual drinking hours, but a pilot program might be limited to Friday and Saturday nights. In those kinds of cities in which mass transit is viable and distances are too great for a full program of subsidized cab rides, it might be possible to plan a "cab and ride" system that combines taxi rides to transit terminals for suburbanites planning to drink in the city.

There are many questions to be answered about the functioning of subsidized alternative transportation programs. Of crucial importance is whether those drivers most likely to consume alcohol in greatly impairing doses would be relatively more or less likely to use cheap taxicabs. Such people are believed to be generally difficult to influence with safety measures—for instance, they fail to fasten their seat belts (Preusser, Williams, and Lund, 1986)—and they may also resist incentives to use alternative transportation. However, these incentives, being of a different order, may be more successful than other policies with this group.

Given the lack of experience and knowledge in this area, it is premature to support the widespread adoption of specific alternative-transportation policies. However, demonstration projects together with evaluation are certainly worth undertaking. A well-conceived pilot study would answer such crucial questions as the extent of use and the cost per trip, as well as savings in lives and serious crashes. In our consideration of possible future demonstration projects concerning drunk driving, a subsidized taxi system during drinking hours would be a far more useful investment in knowledge and prospective policy than yet another police enforcement crackdown or alcohol treatment program.

Designated driver programs

When people go out to drink together, the possibility of designating a driver for the group who will refrain from consuming alcoholic beverages permits combining drinking with private automobile transportation while avoiding drunk driving. Unlike the general subsidized transportation alternatives discussed above, this option has frequently been implemented in recent years. Many of these programs are sponsored by bars, which stand to profit by selling more alcohol to the nondriving members of the party. The latter need not be restrained in their drinking by the danger of having to drive while impaired. Indeed, an advantage from the bar's viewpoint—but a possible disadvantage from the viewpoint of public health—is that total sales to a group with a designated driver may exceed the amount that the group would have purchased in the absence of the policy. At the same time, the bar sponsoring a designated driver program avoids potential liability for highway damage caused by its patrons.

Designated driver programs do not have to be formalized. As Apsler (1989) has noted in reviewing the literature, the concept is adopted informally by people traveling to private parties or to other places where they expect to drink. He cites poll data (158) showing that the concept is supported in the abstract by large majorities of drinkers, who indicate a desire to use such programs and a willingness to take the role of the designated driver. He reports that, in a Boston-area survey, more than half of drivers who also drink stated that they had participated in a group with a designated driver, though only 3 percent said that they were encouraged to designate a nondrinking driver by a bar or restaurant. Snortum, Hauge, and Berger (1986) found, in national surveys, that 12 percent of Americans and 76 percent of Norwegians drinking in groups appointed a nondrinking driver.

Little evaluation of these programs has been published. Given the social desirability of reporting use of designated driver programs, one may suspect that the Snortum, Hauge, and Berger estimates exaggerate this use, at least for the United States. Apsler, Harding, and Goldfein

(1987, summarized in Apsler, 1989) surveyed formal programs, mostly sponsored by bars, and concluded that they were little used. The participating bars implemented the programs by offering free nonalcoholic drinks, food, and coupons for future drinks; the programs were publicized by posters, table tents, and other forms of in- house notification. However, the median number of designated drivers served in participating establishments was fewer than twenty per week, and the researchers estimated that fewer than 10 percent of eligible groups participated in a designated driver program. Solo drinkers, by definition, could not be included, and the program would seldom be meaningful for couples. In addition, logistic considerations (for example, widely separated residences) and group norms of mutuality in drinking were noted among the reasons for the limited appeal of these programs. Apsler concludes, "Based on scanty results, the main effect of publicity about the designated driver tactic may be to encourage drinkers to ride with abstainers or light drinkers when such individuals happen to be available and willing to transport others" (1989: 166).

There seems little reason to expect that further research would contradict the conclusions of Apsler and his colleagues. Designated driver programs may be sensible responses to the dependence of drinkers on private automobile transportation in some cases, and they are approved both by drivers and by representatives of the hospitality industry. For the reasons noted, however, they are unlikely to offer major reductions in drinkers' need to drive. There is the danger that these programs may promote heavy drinking among nondrivers by reducing fears of its consequences, and they may subvert server training programs by purporting to remove one of the strongest reasons for responsible service practices. The programs may be encouraged for what they can accomplish at low cost and in hopes that over time their availability will lead to increased and appropriate use—but expectations that they will bring about major reductions in drunk driving appear unwarranted.

Safe rides programs

Like designated driver programs, safe rides programs allow for collaboration between public health and hospitality industry interests. The fundamental idea is that such programs offer alternative transportation by an alcohol server to a drinker who appears to have consumed a greatly impairing amount. Informally, this is the bartender calling a cab for the intoxicated customer. Such behavior, especially in places like neighborhood taverns where the customers are known to the servers, is part of folklore and has been noted in research (Gusfield, Rasmussen, and Kotarba, 1984). Among the limitations of this technique is that it is very likely applied only to a small percentage of customers who have reached an extreme degree of intoxication and it is unsystematic, dependent on specific situations and personalities. The Samaritan who calls the cab may face a daunting task of convincing needy customers to admit their inadequacy as drinkers and their need for assistance. In the event of success, there remains the problem of returning the customer's car to his home.

Friends can informally provide alternative transportation to intoxicated persons (Hernandez and Rabow, 1987). This practice may be formalized in peer-intervention programs ("Friends don't let friends drive drunk"). In addition, social hosts may invite guests who have imbibed heavily to spend the night, a technique reported by Snortum, Hauge, and Berger (1986) to be quite common in Norway.

Formalized safe rides programs run by taxi companies, hospitals, alcohol-problems groups, and others are frequently found today. Harding, Apsler, and Goldfein (1988) surveyed several hundred such programs and collected detailed data on fifty-two of them. Although several furnished hundreds of free rides per year, the fraction of all possible impaired drivers serviced is doubtless small, for reasons that have already been mentioned in connection with designated driver programs. Perhaps most important, the stereotyped image of the driver who has had sufficient alcohol to be dangerous restricts the operation of safe rides programs to a small, albeit probably extremely dangerous, segment of highly impaired drivers.

Extensive program evaluations are lacking, yet safe rides programs can be endorsed provisionally. They may contribute something to saving lives. Their cost is low—the average for programs surveyed by Harding, Apsler, and Goldfein was less than $12,000 annually—and the programs are popular and seen as useful by the public. In a survey cited by Apsler (1989: 162) nearly eight in ten bar patrons, and nearly nine in ten of the heavy drinkers, indicated they might take advantage of a safe rides service if it were offered. If expectations of results are modest, safe rides programs should be encouraged in the absence of more penetrating but expensive programs such as subsidized alternative transportation. Programs of this type require further study, especially to determine what conditions might foster their greater utilization.

"Contracts for life"

The organization Students Against Driving Drunk (SADD) sponsors a program that arranges contracts between parents and their teenaged children. Children promise to call a parent in the event that they are faced with the need to drive after drinking, and the parent agrees to transport the child on request. Such contracts can be viewed as a family-centered variation of a safe rides program, and most of the comments raised with regard to the general category are likely to apply to some degree in this special case. According to the organization's headquarters, more than five million of these contracts had been signed by 1990. The private nature of the contracts makes evaluation research difficult. The only scientific evaluation of SADD at present is that of Klitzner and others (reported in Klitzner, 1989: 200). This study, described as preliminary, found that the contract appears to increase the number of calls home for a ride, but does not reduce reported drunk driving or riding with a drunk driver. It is hard to explain this disappointing bottom line; the finding begs for further research.

Some critics have noted possible negative consequences of the contract for life. In a private communication, James McKnight expresses the belief that the contract may serve many parents as an assurance that their children will not get in trouble, thus encouraging less parental supervision. The contract for life has also been criticized as implying that teenaged drinking is expected, thus potentially legitimizing it outside of the drinking-and-driving context.

Reducing access to driving

Broad-based prohibitions on driving are a political impossibility in the United States. Acknowledgment of the dependence of nearly everyone on the automobile, along with the political influence of groups with relatively high risks of crash-involvement, has made it difficult to impose stringent safety standards on the licensing of almost any group, for example, the elderly and the visually and physically handicapped. However, narrowly focused driving prohibitions may be feasible as means to reduce drunk driving. A special case is license actions against drivers who have driven while impaired. A more general case concerns driving by young people. Because youth constitute a politically weak segment of society, restriction of their driving, as of their use of alcohol, appears to be feasible where more general prohibitions would not be.

There are reasons beyond political expediency for restricting young people's driving licenses. The principal one is that youths, especially young men, experience extremely high rates of serious and fatal crashes (Williams, 1985; 1987; Fell, 1987). Alcohol and other drugs are involved in disproportionate numbers of these crashes, even though the teens may drink and drive proportionately less than other adults: "Teenagers are less likely than adults to drive after drinking, but their crash risks are higher when they do drink, especially at low and moderate blood alcohol concentrations. . . . Teenage drivers accounted for about 15 percent of all alcohol-related fatal crashes in the United States in 1983 although they were only 7 percent of licensed drivers" (Williams, 1985: 38). That this is not the only justifying factor is revealed by the fact that young men's relative risk of having a fatal crash is higher at eighteen and nineteen—ages at which driving is legal in all states—than at seventeen, and it remains relatively elevated throughout the twenties. Probably the greater involvement of older teenagers in far-flung activities (including gainful employment) and their greater social visibility combine to make a minimum driving age higher than sixteen a political impossibility in most of the United States.

Restraint is necessary in discussing policies that, though likely to be effective, are highly unlikely to be politically acceptable. However, this caution does not prevent recommending raising driving ages currently less than sixteen and increasing restrictions on licenses of youthful drivers. These measures can be justified both as general safety measures and as drunk driving countermeasures. Indeed, specific instances of these policies are in effect and doubtless are helping to control drunk driving today.

Licensing age

At the time of this writing, one state—New Jersey—grants full drivers' licenses to its young people only when they reach age seventeen. The modal age for states to grant full licenses is sixteen, but many of them grant extensive driving privileges (and a few give full licenses) at fifteen. Learners' permits are available to people as young as fourteen and a half years of age in some states.

The fact that sixteen-year-old drivers have the highest serious crash rates per mile driven of all age groups suggests that a raised minimum driving age would reduce the toll of serious crashes. Comparison of the experience of young drivers in New Jersey with that in two nearby states (Connecticut and Massachusetts) that license sixteen-year-olds but otherwise have similar laws for beginning drivers indicates that the higher driving age is beneficial. Using data from the period 1975–80, Williams, Karpf, and Zador (1984) found very few sixteen-year-old drivers involved in fatal crashes in New Jersey. The rate was 4 per 100,000 population, compared to 18 in Massachusetts and 26 in Connecticut. Moreover, the fatal-crash involvement of unlicensed sixteen-year-olds was not higher in New Jersey than in the other states. Although there was some evidence that seventeen-year-old drivers in New Jersey may have had higher crash-involvement rates than seventeen-year-olds in the comparison states owing to their inexperience, the total result in terms of deaths per young person or per licensed young driver greatly favored delayed licensing. In short, New Jersey appears to reap the benefit of a low number of fatal crashes for a year in which other states have considerably higher numbers, and this gain is not wiped out by excessive numbers of crashes later on.

The generalizability of this experience is confirmed in an econometric analysis of data from forty-seven states (Levy, 1990). This study found that driving age was strongly related to fatality rates, but driving experience had only a minor effect. Young drivers, especially those aged fifteen, have a relatively high risk of becoming involved in fatal crashes. The fatalities incurred by this group when licensed are not offset by experience effects.

A relevant international parallel is available in Victoria, Australia, where driving licenses are not granted until age eighteen. This is a higher age limit than in any other Australian state. At one point, critics suggested that Victoria reduce its driving age in order to establish training at a younger age, when safe attitudes are easier to instill, and to separate initiation of drinking from that of driving. However, research stimulated by this suggestion (Drummond, 1986) found that Victoria had not only the lowest rate of licensing among young people, but also the lowest rates of fatal and injurious crashes per licensee of all Australian states.

The fact that, in the United States, New Jersey stands alone in delaying driving age implies that it may not be easy to increase the driving age beyond sixteen in other states. Safety is not the only consideration in the granting of licenses. Adolescents, particularly those as old as sixteen, are not as home-centered as young children, and parents may resent the need to chauffeur their teenagers to a host of activities located beyond walking distance. Moreover, they may prefer that their children be drivers themselves rather than passengers in the vehicles of other, albeit older, teenagers. Even though a national telephone survey in 1985 found that 39 percent of adults (and the same proportion of parents of teenagers) preferred a minimum licensing age of eighteen or higher, perhaps the most practical suggestion would be to increase the age for all driving privileges to sixteen where this is not already the case. Only 2 percent of the national sample of adults preferred fifteen as a minimum driving age, in contrast to the 46 percent who preferred age sixteen and the balance who preferred higher ages yet (Williams and Lund, 1986).

Curfews

As an alternative to prohibiting all driving, young people's involvement in drunk driving might be reduced by restricting their licenses to day-time hours or to times not conducive to drinking. There is empirical evidence to justify such a restriction on the grounds of increased traffic safety. As noted by Williams (1987; 1985), less than 20 percent of the mileage of sixteen-year-olds is driven between 9 P.M. and 6 A.M., yet more than 40 percent of their fatal crashes take place during these hours. The rationale of the curfew is to separate young drivers from the hazards occurring at these times, most notably drinking, while allowing them to gain experience in driving at other, less dangerous times of day.

Several states impose some form of curfew on young or beginning drivers. The most stringent curfew on fully licensed drivers is found in New York, where the licenses of sixteen-year-olds are invalid be-tween 9 P.M. and 5 A.M., as are those of seventeen-year-olds under most circumstances if they have not had formal driver training. Drivers under eighteen are prohibited from driving at any time within New York City.

A study of young drivers in the four states with the most stringent curfews (New York, Pennsylvania, Louisiana, and Maryland) found differences of between 25 and 69 percent from control states in numbers of crashes reported to the police (Preusser, Williams, and Zador, 1984). There was no evidence that these advantages were compensated for by more crashes in noncurfew hours, more non-automobile-related injuries, or more injuries to sixteen-year-olds as passengers. It appeared that the curfew laws not only restrained driving during the dangerous hours but also, by making the license less attractive to young people, reduced the proportion of people getting licensed at early ages and therefore their driving. Curfew laws may thus produce part of the effect intended by raising the minimum licensing age—delaying the appearance on the highways of an exceptionally crash-prone group of drivers.

In addition to being effective in reducing crashes among young people, curfew laws are likely to be politically acceptable. The national survey reported by Williams and Lund (1986) found that nighttime driving curfews for young drivers were approved of by 69 percent of the respondents, including 73 percent of parents of teenagers. It stands to reason that states not presently having nighttime curfews should be urged to consider establishing them as a means of reducing young people's involvement in drunk driving particularly and traffic crashes generally.

Graduated licenses

A more complex set of controls on young people's driving is offered by graduated licensing, in which full permission to drive is not granted at once, but rather is given in stages, provisionally. The stages involve progressively fewer controls and are reached by demonstrations of reliability at prior stages or of ability as indicated in progressively more difficult examinations.

All states have at least some degree of graduated licensing in that they issue learner's permits, allowing driving under restricted circumstances, such as during the day when accompanied by a licensed driver. Graduated or provisional licensing merely introduces additional stages in the process before permitting full driving privileges. Progression through the graduated system may require demonstrating violation-free records over a period of time, a measure designed to encourage safe driving by young people. A model for a graduated licensing program was developed in the 1970s under the aegis of the National Highway Traffic Safety Administration, and some of its provisions were adopted into law in Maryland and in California. The effectiveness of these laws has been evaluated (McKnight, Hyle, and Albrecht, 1983; Hagge and Marsh, 1988). In both states there were significant declines in crashes as well as traffic law violations. One of the more elaborate plans for graduated licenses has been offered by the Road Safety Division of the government of South Australia (O'Connor, 1986). It proposes a four-stage learner's permit. At all stages, and for the first year of the full license, there is zero tolerance for alcohol in the blood of the driver. Other restrictions, progressively removed as the driver advances, include the need to have a licensed adult supervisor at all times, daytime driving only, and a prohibition against carrying passengers. The scheme is proposed to begin at age fifteen on the grounds that people of that age are more receptive to parental supervision and less susceptible to peer pressures than older teenagers.

The Australian proposal is complex, but most of its components seem sensible. The nighttime curfew is likely to be effective in reducing crashes, as noted above. Prohibiting the carrying of passengers other than instructors during the early phases of licensing can be justified as protecting the young driver from distractions as well as from peer pressures to drink and display bravado—a reasonable, if unevaluated, precaution. It would also protect other young people from exposure to crash risks as passengers of young drivers. The zero BAC provision recognizes the greater susceptibility of beginning drivers to having alcohol-related crashes. Moreover, beginning drivers are seldom old enough to drink alcoholic beverages legally, and the license scheme would help support the drinking-age law. Beyond these individual components, the model of a long-term learning process constitutes a legal recognition of social-psychological reality.

It is reasonable to conclude that experimentation with various forms of graduated license systems may yield reductions in violations and casualties among young people, as it did in California and Maryland. A scheme similar to the Australian one has been proposed by Mothers Against Drunk Driving (MADD, 1991), and it deserves full consideration.

Driver training

A theoretically plausible alternative to deferring licensing for young people is driver training. Were this training effective, there would be less reason to be concerned with the mileage incurred by youth, for much of it would merely replace that of others, such as parents, who currently provide transportation to young people unable to drive. Indeed, if parents provide transportation to and from an event, and return home in the interim, automobile mileage may be doubled, compromising gains in safety or other benefits from substituting older for younger drivers.

Safer driving is one of the goals of driver education courses offered in high schools at public expense. As a means of instructing young people in basic driving skills, driver education is a clear success. The licensing rate for young people in jurisdictions providing such education is much higher than that in jurisdictions without the education, although sooner or later nearly everyone in America obtains a license. However, driver education apparently does not reduce the crash rates of young people below what they would have been had they obtained their licenses without these courses, for example, by studying at a commercial driving school or with instruction from a parent or peer. In Williams's words,

Unfortunately, the scientific evidence indicates that in terms of subsequent crash involvement, it does not matter how one learns to drive. That is, high school driver education has little or no effect in reducing crashes per licensed driver. Moreover, offering driver education in high school has been shown to encourage teenagers to become licensed earlier than they otherwise would. The net result is more crashes per capita among teenagers when high school driver education is offered. [1987: 111]

Williams cites research showing that when state support for driver education was withdrawn in Connecticut, resulting in the cancellation of driver education classes in several school districts, crashes in those districts declined, while in those districts continuing the courses with local funds crashes remained high. The model Defensive Driving Course curriculum developed by the National Safety Council has been found in competent evaluations to have no effect on crashes (Lund and Williams, 1985). What is more, a carefully considered model driver education program introduced into a set of Georgia schools, which appeared at first to have at least some short-term effects on postlicensing crashes, turned out on closer examination to be disappointing: "There was some evidence that graduates of the enhanced driver education program were more skilled drivers when licensed than their peers who learned how to drive in other ways, but this did not translate into fewer crashes, probably because attitudes and other factors are more important than driving skills in determining teenagers' crash involvement" (Williams, 1987: 111). These case studies are supported by Levy's (1990) analysis of national data on crash fatalities among teenagers. Although there is a significant negative association between these fatalities and mandatory driver education, it is much smaller than the association with age of licensure. Levy concludes that because driver education may contribute to increased licensing of young people, it is likely to have negative consequences for safety.

The paradoxical positive correlation of driver education with crashes is explained by the fact that driver education is very successful in getting young people licensed, but it is less successful in getting them to drive more safely than their peers. Again quoting Williams (1987: 111), driver education "is one way of learning how to drive, but as presently constituted it adds to the motor vehicle injury problem." In contrast, lives can be saved by delaying the licensing of young people, who form an excessively hazardous category of drivers, especially when they consume alcohol.

Politically effective reasons for licensing young people to drive may exist nevertheless, even though doing so increases highway crashes and fatalities. One argument, not without merit in my mind, is that no one can be a complete participant in American society without being a driver, and it is inequitable to deny this privilege because of age or a characteristic statistically associated with age. The other side of the coin is that being a contemporary American involves exposure to a not insignificant chance of injury or death on the highway, for the driver, his passengers, and other roadway users. Delaying licensing is a scientifically demonstrated way of saving lives, especially those of young people, but whether and to what extent we choose to save these lives in this way is a political question requiring the balancing of consequences.

Restraining driving by apprehended drunk drivers

As I noted in chapter 3, license restriction or revocation is a common element in the package of sanctions imposed on apprehended drunk drivers. Courts routinely restrict or suspend licenses of those they convict, and new administrative procedures remove licenses from apprehended drunk drivers even before conviction. The evidence cited in chapter 3 shows that these measures are effective in reducing subsequent crashes and violations. However, these sanctions operate imperfectly when the sanctioned drivers retain access to their cars.

The imperfect nature of incapacitation by license sanctions has' led to proposals to impound or to confiscate the vehicles of drunk drivers, especially of those found to be driving in violation of license actions. Legislation on this issue has been passed in some states, most notably Minnesota, but the opportunities and mandates are reported to be little used, partly because they are procedurally cumbersome and partly because judges decline to impose these consequences on offenders and their families. If impoundment or confiscation could be more fully implemented, perhaps by administrative rather than judicial procedures, such measures could be useful as a last resort in dealing with drivers who disregard orders banning them from driving.

A less restrictive technique for preventing impaired driving by apprehended drunk drivers is the installation in offenders' cars of ignition interlocks tied to breath-testing devices. This technology, best known in the form of the Guardian Interlock, is designed to prevent operation of the vehicle if the driver's breath contains a concentration of alcohol higher than that permitted. Interlock devices are currently being used in many jurisdictions, usually as a condition of probation for convicted drunk drivers. The convicted drivers must generally bear the cost of installing and maintaining the machines on their cars in exchange for the granting of limited driving privileges. Recently, in several Oregon counties, interlocks have been required for the first six months for all new licensees at the termination of judicially imposed revocations. Although the current devices can be thwarted, initial evaluations give hope that impaired driving by known offenders can be significantly reduced through the use of ignition interlocks (e.g., Morse and Elliott, 1990). Interlock installation may obviate the need for extreme incapacitative measures such as long-term incarceration of the offenders or confiscation of family vehicles. Another technological device that promises to help enforce the conditions of probation by monitoring the times of automobile use is the Autotimer. Its effectiveness is currently being evaluated (Voas, 1988b).

Measures like ignition interlocks and time recorders share with treatment and education programs for apprehended drunk drivers the important limitation of being unable to affect directly the behavior of the unapprehended. There are no serious proposals to install interlocks on the entire American automotive fleet. Rather, these are mandated only for known offenders, perhaps even only for those with multiple offenses on their driving records. Since the majority of drivers involved in alcohol-related fatal crashes are not previously known to the authorities, such devices would be incapable of directly affecting the bulk of the drunk driving problem even if they worked perfectly—which, of course, they do not.

It is more difficult to implement policies aimed at reducing driving than those aimed at reducing drinking. Although many parallel techniques are available to apply to both goals, including prohibitions among narrowly defined population segments, price-based disincentives to use, and controls over marketing, we are less willing to apply them to the goal of reducing driving. Indeed, the legitimacy of the attempt to reduce driving in America may be challenged in principle.

Alcohol-policy countermeasures are legitimized by the ambivalent place of drinking in American society. Historically, society has recognized both good and bad aspects of drinking, and the balance has shifted over time, at one point to the degree of near-total prohibition of production and sale of alcoholic beverages. Although experience led us to abandon that approach, we are committed in principle to the need to regulate alcohol. The issue is merely to what degree and by what means.

In contrast, America's love affair with the automobile knows few bounds. The beloved has been noted on occasion to have some blemishes: it has so greatly contributed to congestion that it mocks its own promise of freedom of travel; it has produced so much trash, filth, effluent on the ground and in the air that its owners are impeded in finding the better world the vehicle has promised; and it has annually "sacrificed" tens of thousands of lives in crashes. However, the vast majority of us continue to hold it dear, to value its use and ownership, and to regard its blemishes as minor in comparison with its virtues.

Moreover, transformations wrought by the automobile in the physical structure of the community make reduced driving increasingly difficult to achieve. It is hard to envisage an alternative means of circulation in the relatively dispersed settlement patterns that constitute the fabric of modern metropolises. In the American democracy, it can be meaningfully said that the right to drive is more important than the right to vote.

Transportation policy–based measures aimed at saving lives must therefore be less ambitious than those based in alcohol policy. This does not mean they should be disregarded. However, practical measures of this kind tend to be narrow and compromised. Such broader approaches as large increases in the fuel taxes would be unpopular and politically infeasible. The most appealing of transportation policies would be to render driving less risky through training, but this goal does not appear to be well attained through present programs. Their impact on safety is actually negative because of their success at licensing young people, who are more hazardous drivers than average.

Measures that provide alternative transportation, especially to people who are visibly impaired by drinking, are politically acceptable but have not been widely used. More general countermeasures of this type, such as subsidized taxis, have seldom been considered, even on a trial basis. If we are serious about saving lives, the time has come to undertake these sorts of initiatives to see what in fact can be accomplished with determination and resources.

The greatest demonstrated success in reducing drunk driving with transportation policy as well as alcohol policy has been through limited prohibitions. Although not completely successful in averting exposure to drinking and driving, they are associated with important reductions in crashes among the targeted populations. Indeed, the prohibition approach that delays legal driving appears to be proportionately even more successful in saving lives than that delaying legal drinking. Very few people under the driving age are found driving, whereas many under the legal drinking age are found drinking. The example of New York and other states indicates that curfews on young drivers save lives. New Jersey's curfew shows, further, that total prohibitions on driving up to age seventeen are both practicable and effective in saving lives. Poll data confirm that some such measures are politically acceptable. Their adoption seems a reasonable proposal for saving lives lost and reducing injuries from drunk driving and other sources of crashes.

Saving Lives in Spite of Drunk Driving

My review thus far has been confined to policies designed to reduce the number of miles driven by impaired drivers. Here I look at a different opportunity for policy: reducing injury and saving lives notwithstanding the continued existence of impaired driving. The importance of this approach is underlined by the fact that, although deliberate policies and other factors may reduce it, drunk driving will not and cannot be eliminated as an aspect of a recognizable American society. It bears repeating that its fundamental institutional causes are acceptance of drinking as a leisure activity and commitment to driving as the virtually unique means of transportation in our country, and that elimination of these aspects of the American life-style would be an unrealistic goal.

The continued prevalence of drunk driving, however, can be countered with policies that reduce consequential deaths and injuries. These policies are recommended not as alternatives to those aimed at reducing drunk driving, but as supplements. In my opinion, they are essential parts of an overall package of policies designed to affect the bottom line of deaths and injuries suffered in crashes, including those in which alcohol is a factor.

This approach to saving lives follows the lead of William Haddon (1972). He challenged the road safety establishment of his day (and ours) with the view that "the overriding societal issue in this field is the reduction of losses in damaged people and property that makes it of concern, and that one does not get to a systematic approach in research or in programmes, or do all

6

one can, if one only talks about preventing crashes" (2). Although I categorize the various countermeasures differently from him, I am inspired by his understanding that conditions during and after crashes are as crucial to the outcome as those preceding crashes and that policies reducing the occurrence of crashes must be supplemented by policies reducing their consequences. To quote Haddon again,

The single most important and essential point . . . is that the emphasis, the priorities, placed upon given loss-reduction countermeasures among the options available must be based on their effectiveness in reducing the end-results in damage—not necessarily in preventing the initiation of the events themselves. This frequently means that primary emphasis, if rationally selected, must be placed on other than pre-event countermeasures. [1972, 4]

He continues with such examples as providing a safety net for the acrobat rather than (or in addition to) preaching safe performance and properly wrapping items to be mailed rather than exhorting postal employees not to drop packages.

This approach is characterized by an emphasis on technology, rather than on education, training, and therapy. In the words of Haddon's former colleague, Leon Robertson (1980: 13), "Engineering for people rather than trying to engineer people by changing their behaviors has the better record of success. Injury control programs that automatically protect people without their having to take any action are the most successful."

The policies discussed in this chapter are directed toward attenuating the links in the causal chain connecting impaired driving with injuries and deaths. The first set of policies concerns the link between impairment and error: if the driving task can be sufficiently simplified or the capabilities of the driver or vehicle sufficiently enhanced, it may be possible to compensate to some degree for impairment and thus reduce the numbers of consequential errors. The second set concerns the link between error and crashes: if hazards can be removed from the environment or restrained in their capacity to inflict damage, crashes can be eliminated or made less severe. The third set concerns the link between crashes and injuries: if people can be protected from crash forces they are less likely to be injured, and the injuries experienced will be less severe. The fourth set of policies is directed at the link between injuries and death: if effective care can be promptly provided to the injured, they are less likely to die as a consequence of their injuries. The causal chain underlying this exposition is diagrammed in the following figure:

Impairment → Error → Crash → Injury → Death

Attenuating each of these links offers a promising means of saving lives.

Lifesaving policies of the type discussed in this chapter, although they are proposed on the basis of concern with alcohol-related crashes and are especially effective in dealing with deaths experienced in those crashes, have the advantage of being applicable to the reduction of injuries and deaths caused by factors other than alcohol. Highways designed to lessen the possibility of traffic conflicts, roadsides free of unnecessary hazards, vehicles that cushion their occupants from crash forces, and facilities for providing prompt medical assistance in emergencies have very broad benefits. Although impaired drivers and passengers in their vehicles may benefit disproportionately from such measures, these amenities and services increase the safety of drivers and passengers (that is, nearly all Americans) in general. The generality of these benefits should be considered in determining the cost effectiveness of policies adopted because of their impact on deaths due to drunk driving.

Addressing the link between impairment and error

An impaired driver is less able than an unimpaired one to perform the tasks required for a safe trip. The impaired driver is less alert and competent. Perception, judgment, and execution of decisions are less accurate and efficient in an impaired driver. Other things being equal, impaired drivers commit more errors, experience more crashes, and suffer more injuries and death. However, the consequences of impairment differ depending on the difficulty of the task presented. A simpler task results in fewer errors. The benefits of simplicity accrue to all but are most significant for the impaired. They can go a long way toward neutralizing the safety risks associated with alcohol. (Although I write concerning driving impairment by alcohol, impairment can be produced by other drugs, fatigue, old age, and other factors.)

An important means of reducing the complexity and difficulty of driving is to prevent or moderate the conflict of streams of traffic. This is achieved in an obvious manner through the construction of freeways, which replace intersections with ramps and merging lanes, permitting the smooth integration of traffic with minimal need to adjust speed and direction in order to avoid colliding with other vehicles. The classic example is the Interstate highway system. That system has mileage-based crash rates less than half those prevailing on the rural highway system it replaced. In 1987, the Interstate fatal crash rate was 1.27 per 100 million vehicle miles traveled, compared with 3.10 for other federal-aid primary highways (Federal Highway Administration, 1988). This despite the fact that the Interstates carry traffic at higher average speeds and that therefore the risk of death in a given crash is higher. Although some of this advantage may relate to different types of traffic on the Interstates and to reduction of roadside hazards, some of it is almost certainly due to the less demanding nature of driving on a limited-access highway. The effect of the low Interstate rates on general crash rates is significant, for although Interstate highways in 1989 accounted for fewer than thirty-five thousand miles of roads—less than 1 percent of the nation's rural highway network—they carried about a fifth of all rural highway mileage and accounted for about 10 percent of the total miles traveled on all public streets and roads in the United States (Federal Highway Administration, 1989). Although it is fanciful and impracticable to envisage unlimited expansions of the freeway system, the impact of additional construction on the death rate is likely to be major. Moreover, the beneficial effect of simplifying the driving task in this way is probably disproportionately effective in avoiding collisions in which the driver is impaired.

This enthusiasm requires tempering because the impact of freeway construction on the actual numbers of deaths experienced is usually, owing to the increased traffic generated by better roads, less than expected on the basis of crash rates. In other words, some of the safety benefits are transformed into increased mobility. Furthermore, limited-access highways experience a unique kind of alcohol-related hazardous behavior, that of driving in the wrong direction (with no easy escape route). This problem is addressed in many places through the use of wrong-way signs, the effectiveness of which might be increased if they were larger and better lighted.

The driving task can be made easier by engineering interventions less comprehensive than the building of freeways. Examples include providing generous lane widths, signalizing busy intersections, and providing adequate drainage for the roadway (Retting, 1991). The fact that the typical single-vehicle fatality involving alcohol involves running off the road at a curve suggests the utility of straightening curves as a drunk-driving countermeasure.

An alternative and far cheaper approach to simplifying the driving task is to provide the driver with better information about highway hazards. The basis of this approach to reducing errors by impaired drivers is that "drivers with elevated blood alcohol contents receive less visual information, and that information which is received is processed more slowly as a result of the other effects of alcohol ingestion" (Editorial, 1980: 13). Although this approach may be promising, it is difficult to come to precise estimations of its potential. Calculations by an engineer for Mercedes-Benz suggest considerable importance for even slight decreases in the time in which evasive action is taken in a pending collision: "[R]oughly half of all collisions between vehicles could be prevented if each driver would initiate his accident avoiding maneuver approximately a half to one second earlier" (Enke, 1979: 789). In addition, according to this source, "[b]etter visibility and better recognizability of the course of a road and the traffic on the road by correct configuration . . . and elimination of view-impairing obstacles are important long-term measures for an earlier recognition of the traffic situations by the users" (801). Although these particular calculations—apparently the only ones in the literature— appear to lack an adequate empirical base, and the claims made for potential benefits of as little as a half-second seem intuitively to be overwrought, the general proposition that advance information about hazards may reduce their toll seems reasonable. The Federal Highway Administration has endorsed the effectiveness of roadway markers and delineators as hazard mitigators and of improved sight distance (leveling and straightening roads) and illumination, among other measures, as means for reducing fatal multivehicle crashes (Nichols and Shinar, 1990).

Examples of measures intended to reduce crashes by providing more information to drivers about the road include chevron markers on curves, lines and posts to delineate the edge of the highway, and standard warning and speed advisory signs before curves. A survey of state highway departments in 1982 found that use of these devices was common and that highway officials generally believed in their effectiveness but that formal evaluations were rare, and evidence concerning effectiveness was mainly subjective (Wright, Hall, and Zador, 1983).

It may be that at least in some situations the drivers' need for this information is intuitively obvious, and the cost of providing it is modest in comparison. However, wise policy requires that considerably more be known before specific technology can be advocated with confidence in its cost-effectiveness.

An apparent reduction in nighttime crashes was found in a study of the effects of reflectorized markers installed in the center lines of Georgia roads with relatively sharp curves. The study found that the ratio of nighttime to daytime crashes declined by 22 percent (Zador, Wright, and Karpf, 1982). Moreover, the effect was 12 percent greater among single-vehicle crashes, suggesting greater effectiveness for impaired drivers. A broader attempt to evaluate provision of various curve-delineation markers found evidence that nighttime speeds on curves shifted upward when the curves were marked, indicating that drivers may have felt better oriented; greater safety is among the possible inferences, but no crash information was provided in the report (Zador et al., 1987).

Pavement edge line marking is especially interesting because of its low cost. In experimental studies, painted edge lines were varied from nonexistent to eight inches in width. It was found that edge lines of any width improved the performance of unimpaired drivers on curves and that drivers dosed with alcohol to 0.05 percent or 0.08 percent BAC drove better with wide edge lines than with narrow ones or none at all (Nedas, Balcar, and Macy, 1982). However, sponsorship of the research by a manufacturer of pavement marking material taints the findings, and confidence in the utility of this simple, cheap measure has been eroded by findings from a study in New Mexico, where edge lines of different widths were painted on randomly selected hazardous road segments. Crashes were not reduced in the segments with "better" markings (Hall, 1987). Similarly, fatal crashes were not lower on highways with raised lane markings, according to a study based on FARS data (Shinar and Fell, 1990). Although it is premature to write off the potential of edge lining and other economical means of providing more information to drivers (Ward, 1987), endorsement of specific techniques must be guarded pending better evaluation of those widely used at present. For instance, chevron curve markers are employed in all states, and their design, use, and spacing in the future might best be based on evaluations of experience to date.

The link between impairment and error can also be addressed by using and improving available vehicle technologies. The consequences of impairment can be reduced to the extent that decisions are removed from the driver and allocated to the vehicle. A current example is antilock brakes, which substitute computer-programmed controls to prevent skidding for a driver control procedure that is unusually difficult and frequently botched. To the extent that impaired drivers do worse in demanding tasks such as controlling a skid, they should be relatively more helped by this technology. Although there has been little field research verifying its safety accomplishments, the technology is endorsed by laboratory studies and has been well received in the market. In the near future, innovations such as devices warning the driver of a threatening hazard and automatic speed control and braking linked to radar detection of a collision course are possible (Enke, 1979; Treat, 1980; Schwing, 1987):

> Sensor systems could be utilized for the detection of vehicles in the blind spot and back-up warning when a car engages reverse. . . . Semi-automatic maintenance of a driver-set distance between the host vehicle and the car ahead during cruise-control operation, known as headway control, could be another safety feature. Collision warning systems could provide for the surveillance of the space around the vehicle and warn of potential or imminent collisions from any direction. A collision mitigation system could be enabled before an unavoidable collision and automatically enhance occupant protection from a collision coming from any direction. [Walsh, 1991: 23–24]

Full automation of driving is the ultimate step in implementing intelligent vehicle-highway systems, but this, if at all possible, will be attained in the distant future.

In sum, impairment can be countered with interventions that reduce the likelihood of consequent error. Simplifying the driving task through highway modification, providing better information for drivers, and increasing the competence of the vehicle through technology are examples. To the extent that these are effective, it is possible to attain safety even in the presence of driver impairment. This is not to argue for complacency with regard to the impairment, but rather to urge inclusion of the interventions mentioned in the overall approach to saving lives lost to drunk driving.

Addressing the link between error and crashes

Even though impairment causes driver errors, crashes are not an inevitable consequence. The error may be corrected or the crash outcome avoided. Part of the safety advantage of Interstate highways over typical rural roads doubtless lies in the wide lanes and typical broad, grassy median separations that more easily allow correction of driving errors, whether these are caused by impairment or lack of skill, inexperience, or other factors. Additionally, a vehicle running off such a road is much more likely to come to a stop without impacting other vehicles or fixed objects, that is, without experiencing a crash. This understanding leads to suggestions for saving lives on all kinds of roads.

The likelihood of avoiding a crash, given driver error, depends in large part on characteristics of the highway environment. A recent review of data on crash-related fatalities from the FARS accident reporting system and other places noted that nearly three in ten fatal crashes in 1988 involved collisions with roadside hazards (IIHS Facts, 1989). More than half the drivers killed in these collisions had BACs in excess of 0.10 percent. The most frequently struck object—involved in a quarter of roadside-hazard fatal crashes—was a tree. Other common factors in these fatalities included poles, such as utility standards and light posts; guardrails and other traffic barriers; ditches and embankments; and curbs and culverts. The role of these hazards was found to be most pronounced in single-vehicle running-off-the-road crashes, which are especially likely to involve alcohol-impaired driving.

Such crashes can be reduced by modifying the environment, removing obstacles from the vicinity of the roadway. For instance, Perchonok et al. (1978) found, in a study of run-off-the-road crashes, that the frequency of collisions with wooden utility poles declines by approximately 5 percent for every six feet of distance between the poles and the roadway. Inasmuch as this type of crash is relatively likely to involve impaired drivers, removal of poles, trees, and other hazards from the immediate vicinity of roads could be among the more effective measures currently available to reduce deaths associated with drunk driving.

Addressing the link between crashes and injury

Perhaps the most important lifesaving opportunities available today lie in the area of attenuating the consequences of crashes. Even though impairment results in errors and crashes, lives can be spared if the forces experienced in the crashes are reduced to levels that can be tolerated by the human body. Although someone who has experienced a stubbed toe in a three-mile-per-hour collision with the bathroom door at night may be skeptical, a properly packaged vehicle occupant can survive far more severe collisions with little or no injury. Much of the opportunity in this area lies in providing and using protective technology, including such devices as child restraints, helmets for motorcyclists, seat belts for occupants of vehicles, and automatic restraints, including air bags. These devices all recognize the possibility of crashes; they operate not by reducing crashes, but by reducing the severity of the forces applied to the body in the course of crash events. Their effectiveness is achieved notwithstanding the existence of drunk driving and other causes of crashes.

Before I consider the issues surrounding this technology, it should be noted that some of the highway modifications discussed in the prior section may have the effect of reducing the severity of crashes, rather than avoiding them. A collision with a guardrail is counted as a roadside-hazard crash, but such a collision is preferable to one involving the bridge abutment or cliff that lies beyond. The roadside-hazard collision with a median barrier is almost certainly preferable to a head-on collision with another vehicle in the opposite lane. Technology can be applied to install a replaceable light post that collapses on impact in preference to one that remains unscathed at the expense of the occupants of a colliding vehicle. These examples have in common the substitution of moderate decelerations for sharp and sudden ones, with consequent reductions in the forces experienced by vehicle occupants and thus in injuries produced.

The potential for saving lives

A variety of state and federal safety standards applied to automobiles since the mid-1960s has mandated the introduction of injury-reducing technology into the vehicle fleet. Such features as steering columns that absorb energy in crashes rather than impaling the drivers, windshields that resist penetration, reinforcement of roofs and doors, removal of potentially injurious knobs and buttons, and padding of surfaces likely to be impacted in crashes appear to have made a difference.

The costs and benefits of federal standards for protecting passenger car occupants were surveyed by the U.S. General Accounting Office

(1976), based on data from New York and North Carolina. Actual crash data were compared with projections based on experience from years before the issuance of standards by either the General Services Administration, charged with federal procurement, or the National Highway Safety Bureau, charged with responsibility for vehicle safety standards. The report estimated that standards issued between 1966 and 1970 had reduced fatalities by more than twenty-eight thousand from 1966 through 1974, at a cost of $7.2 billion.

The impact of these standards was also evaluated by Robertson (1981), using a correlational analysis of the FARS data file from 1975 through 1978. Occupant death rates were substantially lower in cars produced in years when the most stringent standards came into effect. Robertson estimated that in the four-year period he studied, the federal regulations had prevented thirty-seven thousand deaths. Moreover, "[t]he death reductions associated with federal regulations were found among pedestrians, bicyclists, and motorcyclists in collisions with regulated cars as well as occupants of those cars, providing no support for the theory that occupant death reductions were offset by increased risk to pedestrians or other nonoccupants of the regulated cars" (1981: 821).

Robertson's methods and estimate have been criticized (see Evans, 1991: 81–83), but his general point receives support from other studies. Econometric methods were employed by the Brookings Institution staff (Crandall, et al., 1986) in a study estimating a reduction in fatalities of about 30 percent from statistical projections of what would otherwise have been the case: "Had automobiles been as unsafe in 1981 as in 1965, the estimates... suggest that total fatalities would have been 18,000 to 22,000 above their actual 1981 level" (69). This reduction was accomplished at an estimated cost for both safety and pollution regulations of between $2,222 and $2,532 per vehicle, with safety accounting for between 30 and 39 percent ($667 and $987, respectively) of the cost (39).

An economist with the U.S. Office of Management and Budget has undertaken a comparison of the lifesaving achievements of safety regulations with those of regulations pertaining to other health risks, especially cancer (Morrall, 1986). He notes that the accomplishments of a regulation relate not only to its effectiveness in reducing injuries given an accident/crash, but also to the degree of risk posed by the hazard addressed. Thus, even a highly effective regulation if addressed to a minuscule risk might not yield much of an accomplishment. Looking at twenty-six final rules from a variety of federal agencies charged with regulating work and product safety, environmental pollution, the quality of food and drugs, and safety on the roads, rails, and in the air, Morrall concludes that the auto safety regulations are by far the most important:

A very large share of the regulatory benefits of the rules that were issued—4030 lives saved annually, or 75 percent of the benefits of all final rules—was due to just four regulations, all dealing with motor vehicle design. These were the NHTSA's collapsible steering column requirement, its passive restraint rule requiring air bags or automatic seat belts, and its standards for fuel system integrity and side-door strength. In contrast, the [Environmental Protection Agency] has issued just one rule estimated to save a large number of lives, which is its ban of trihalomethanes (chloroform and other organics in drinking water), estimated to save 322 lives annually. The other six final rules issued by the EPA save an estimated five lives per year *in total*. [29]

The NHTSA regulations are also judged to be cost-effective, that is, to produce estimated savings amounting to more than their costs. Costs per life saved range between $100,000 and $1.3 million for the safety rules mentioned, compared with more than $19 million (and as much as $72 billion) per life saved as a result of the ten least cost-effective of the twenty-six final rules reviewed by Morrall.

That there is still room for safety contributions from basic vehicle design is indicated by the recent finding, in a study of British coroners' records, that 44 percent of fatalities in side-impact crashes might have been prevented with existing technology. Among the study's specific recommendations were stronger vehicle side structures and more energy-absorbing padding (Lestina, Gloyns, and Rattenbury, 1990).

The FARS data file has lent itself to a sophisticated technique for investigating the effect of specific design features. The method, devised by Leonard Evans (1986; 1991), has been applied in numerous articles by Evans and other researchers. Briefly, it compares the ratio of deaths among protected occupants to those of unprotected occupants in the same vehicle, and controls this comparison with the ratio of deaths among unprotected occupants in the same seating positions.

For example, to estimate the effect of seat belts, the ratio of belted drivers killed to unbelted passengers killed is controlled by the ratio of unbelted drivers killed to unbelted passengers killed. The latter ratio reflects differences in the dangerousness of the seating positions. The former ratio divided by the latter estimates the savings introduced by the belts. The addition of other statistical controls permits different estimates by age, sex, and other occupant characteristics.

Using this method, Evans (1988) has estimated the effectiveness in preventing deaths of wearing three-point seat belts (providing both lap and shoulder restraints) at about 43 percent for front-seat occupants of cars and about 18 percent for rear-seat occupants. For motorcyclists, the lifesaving results of helmets are estimated to be about 27 percent. Although engineering laboratory tests simulating fairly severe crashes have suggested even greater potential effects, these may not be realized in the field because, among other reasons, some crashes are of such extreme severity that no reductions achievable through restraints could reasonably be expected to save lives, and many others are so minor that even unprotected occupants will be uninjured. However, although it is possible to disagree with Evans's estimates in detail, it is hard to disagree with him that "[f]atality reductions of the magnitudes found for any of these devices would be viewed as major achievements if they were associated with a new medical procedure or drug" (1987: 13).

Evans's estimate of the effectiveness of motorcycle helmets in reducing crash deaths is confirmed by an independent estimate of 29 percent based on the same technique applied to a broader data base by NHTSA staff (Wilson, 1989). The NHTSA estimates that, because they wore helmets, 4,645 motorcyclists' lives were saved between 1982 and 1987; had helmet-wearing been universal, more than 9,000 lives would have been saved.

The NHTSA staff obtained even more promising estimates of the effectiveness of automobile front-seat lap and shoulder belts by applying Evans's method to FARS data between 1982 and 1985 (Partyka, 1988a). Depending on the year, the estimates ranged between 43 and 56 percent.

Perhaps the most effective devices for saving lives through reducing crash forces are safety seats for infants and young children. In a highly persuasive study, Partyka (1988b) derived estimates of lives saved by applying the Evans method to FARS data for 1982 through 1987. These indicate that the devices produced a 69 percent reduction in fatalities of infants (under one year of age) and 47 percent among children aged one through four. Further, inasmuch as some of the devices were doubtless improperly used and therefore less effective than they might have been, the potential for improvement is higher than these estimates suggest. Chuck Hurley of the Insurance Institute for Highway Safety stated in a *Newsweek* article of January 14, 1991, "Car seats are virtually a vaccine against the leading cause of death to kids." Unfortunately, they are used in fewer than a third of reported fatal crashes, a matter than can be considered a shocking waste of opportunity.

The usage problem

As the last example pointedly illustrates, the principal challenge and opportunity for lifesaving in the area of the linkage between crashes and injury is to increase the use of presently available technology, specifically seat belts, motorcycle helmets, and child restraint devices. The level of seat belt use in the early 1980s was estimated at less than 15 percent (Goodell-Grivas, cited in Stutts, Hunter, and Campbell, 1984). Repeated confirmation of the effectiveness of the devices, along with their universal installation and ease of attachment, makes this nonuse appear irrational. This impression is supported by the empirical falsehood of many beliefs expressed about the devices, for instance, that they are likely to trap a driver in a burning car (O'Day and Filkins, 1983). Nonuse of seat belts appears to be tied to the same factors that effectively impede preventive behavior in the health field more generally: a disinclination to attend to very low-probability events, and the desire to show tangible returns on expenses (Slovic, Fischhoff, and Lichtenstein, 1978). The effort required to use the devices properly, though small, is not rewarded with obvious gains.

Most of the research on nonuse of protective devices concerns seat belts. Seat belt use is estimated primarily through surveys that link use and nonuse to opinions and personal characteristics. This approach, however, has a serious shortcoming. Since seat belt use is socially desirable (Wagenaar, Streff, and Maybee, 1987), responses about use are likely to be exaggerated in surveys, as they are in Harris's finding that 63 percent of persons reported using them in 1989 (Highway and Vehicle Safety Report, 1990). More accurate estimates come from field studies in which use is observed and recorded by the researchers (e.g., Preusser, Williams, and Lund, 1986).

Research finds that failure to attach seat belts is associated with low levels of education and income. The least-educated and the poorest people are least likely to use their belts and thus most likely to suffer disproportionately from deaths and injuries in crashes (Campbell and Campbell 1988, 47–48; O'Day and Filkins, 1983). Younger drivers are less likely to wear belts than are older ones, and, most significantly, drinking drivers are less likely to wear them than nondrinkers. In their observational study in southeastern New York State, Preusser, Williams, and Lund (1986) found that drivers leaving bars were much more likely to be unbelted than a comparable group of non-bargoers during both nighttime and daytime hours. What is more, they found belt use to be correlated with the size and recency of the vehicle— usage was greater in larger and newer vehicles, perhaps reflecting the age and financial status of their owners.

Information campaigns

It is plausible that irrational behaviors might be countered if the public were well informed of the reasons for using seat belts. Slovic, Fischhoff, and Lichtenstein (1978) found in laboratory experiments that subjects could be persuaded to purchase insurance against rare threats by encouraging them to think in a longer time perspective, that is, to evaluate the risk of being involved in a crash in the course of a lifetime rather than on the next trip. However, there is little evidence that providing information for the purpose of encouraging seat belt use is effective in the real world. Williams and Lund (1988: 52), following a review of the relevant literature, state, "Seat belt education may have some positive benefits in creating a climate that facilitates passage of belt use laws, but it has not worked to increase seat belt use directly in the United States or in other countries."

A classical experiment was conducted by Robertson et al. (1974) in a West Virginia town with a cable television system wired to permit marketing studies. Promotional messages (some of which later won awards for their quality) were delivered to an experimental set of households and withheld from a matched control set. Observers were placed to record the use and nonuse of seat belts by drivers along with vehicle license numbers, permitting analysis for the opportunity to receive the messages. The average television watcher was estimated to have viewed one of the messages two or three times per week. A national campaign on this scale would have cost about $7 million in 1972 dollars.

The campaign was totally without effect. Seat belt wearing was the same, whether the car belonged to an experimental household, a control household, or a household lacking cable television. Seat belt use in the community for some reason declined during the course of the experiment (from levels in the midteens to 10 percent or less), but the decline was experienced in all groups and was neither retarded nor accelerated by the message campaign. This definitive study, then, like the prior literature reviewed there, offers no encouragement to warrant an investment in media messages as a means to increase the use of automobile seat belts.

Mandatory use laws

Laws mandating the use of vehicle safety devices were initially adopted in the United States for child restraints in cars and crash helmets for motorcycle riders. Laws mandating the use of helmets were at one point enacted by forty-seven states, in part because of federal threats to withhold highway construction funds from those that did not. The laws produced near universal use of these protective devices by motorcyclists and resulted in major reductions in cyclist fatality rates in the states that adopted them (Watson, Zador, and Wilks, 1981). When in 1976 Congress prohibited the secretary of transportation from withholding funds for states failing to mandate helmet laws—and some states consequently repealed their legislation—helmet use fell and casualties rose (U.S. Department of Transportation, 1980; Berkowitz, 1981).

Laws mandating the use of child restraints were adopted in all states by the mid-1980s. Evaluations found that the laws were followed by important increases in the proportions of restrained children and decreases in the rates of injuries and fatalities (Wagenaar and Webster, 1985). Meanwhile, initial reports from Australia, Britain, and other jurisdictions demonstrated the ability of mandatory seat belt use laws to reduce the number of lives lost on the highway (see Mackay, 1985).

Experience with laws mandating use of occupant restraints in vehicles provides perhaps unexpected evidence of the effectiveness of safety measures premised on changing the behavior of individuals. This approach had been deemphasized in the United States, in favor of vehicle and highway engineering measures, ever since federal leadership in safety policy was established with the creation of the U.S. Department of Transportation (Mashaw and Harfst, 1990). However, reports of lives saved owing to mandatory seat belt use laws abroad were followed by adoption of such laws in many American jurisdictions. The first of these was passed by New York in 1984, and similar statutes were soon enacted in most states. The legislation was favored with lobbying by auto companies, following modification of Federal Motor Vehicle Safety Standard 208 to provide that if mandatory seat belt wearing laws were not widely adopted by the states, automobile manufacturers would have to install passive restraints in their vehicles.

The laws adopted by the various states differ considerably in their details, including the conditions under which a violator can be cited. In most states, a citation for violating the seat belt law can be issued only in conjunction with one for another traffic law violation; thus, the fact that a motorist is observed unbelted cannot by itself justify a ticket. This rule, which permits only what is called secondary enforcement, is unusual in world perspective. Most countries, but only a minority of American states, permit primary enforcement of seat belt laws, whereby police are authorized to stop motorists and issue citations for driving while unbelted (Williams and Lund, 1988).

The use or nonuse of seat belts (especially the three-point ones, which cross the chest), like that of motorcycle helmets, is generally a simple matter for police to observe in the course of their routine patrols, and the laws are therefore relatively easy to enforce. In deterrence theory terms, the likelihood of apprehension for violators can be made very high, which leads to the expectation that determined enforcement of these laws should result in large increments of compliance. This should be the case particularly when enforcement is not impeded by the requirement that it be secondary to enforcement of other laws. The expectation is confirmed in studies of belt use, of crash-related fatalities, and of injuries.

Although, as a result of procurement standards, seat belts have been installed in all new vehicles sold in the United States since 1966, initial use rates were low, seldom exceeding 25 percent of drivers. This was true despite the relatively small effort required to attach and wear them and the campaigns of safety organizations to promote their use. Reviewing the evaluation literature, Williams and Lund (1988: 57–58) offered the following summary of the effects of mandatory use laws on seat belt usage:

1. Use rates increased in states that passed laws, from very low levels before the laws went into effect to between 40 and 60 percent right after.

2. The typical pattern is that the highest use rates are achieved immediately after the laws go into force—that is, in the first month— followed by declines within a few months and eventual stabilization [at a level higher than initially prevailed] . . .

3. There are substantial state-to-state variations in usage rates . . .

4. The variation in experience for different states relates strongly to whether the law can be enforced on a primary or secondary basis and to how vigorously the law is enforced. States with primary enforcement provisions have experienced the largest increases in use rates.

Usage also seems to be related to the severity of the penalty for nonuse. Again, theory would predict this, given what appears to be reasonable levels of perceived certainty of punishment for nonusers of belts. For example, the North Carolina law was introduced in stages. In the first year, between October 1985 and November 1986, police issued only warning tickets. Belt use before the law, observed by researchers, was in the neighborhood of 25 percent. It rose to between 40 and 50 percent during the warning phase. In January 1987 police began to issue formal citations, punishable with a $25 fine: observed belt use rose to 78 percent. It subsequently stabilized at about 60 percent, in conformity with the general pattern noted by Williams and Lund (Reinfurt et al., 1988).

The responsiveness of belt use rates to enforcement has been demonstrated in publicized police crackdowns on nonuse. Examples include campaigns in Ottawa, Canada, and Elmira, New York. These campaigns are easier to launch in jurisdictions that have laws permitting primary enforcement, but a campaign in Modesto under California's secondary-enforcement law also showed an important increase in belt use (Williams and Lund, 1988: 64–66).

The mandatory use laws often exclude certain groups of people at risk, especially those in the rear seats of automobiles and people riding in pickup trucks and vans, and vehicle occupants in excluded categories are less likely than those specified in the law to use their belts (Wells, Williams, and Fields, 1989) However, some observers (e.g., Wagenaar and Wiviott, 1985) have noted a spillover effect from mandatory use laws, with greater belt usage among vehicle occupants not directly covered by the laws than among similarly situated vehicle occupants in jurisdictions lacking the laws.

Mandatory use laws have been shown to produce savings of lives. This has been demonstrated with interrupted time-series analyses that have found fatality declines precisely coincident with the inception of the laws (e.g., Lund, Zador, and Pollner, 1987) as well as econometric analyses of multistate data (Skinner and Hoxie, 1988). However, typical estimates of the effect of the laws on fatalities lie between 5 and 15 percent, a far smaller change than expected given the typically large increases in usage levels. The failure of fatalities to decline in proportion to increases in belt use is partly explained by the fact that vehicle occupants who are most likely to be involved in crashes commonly conform least to the belt use laws. Examples are teenagers, speeders, and drinking drivers (Williams and Lund, 1988: 59). This situation has been noted even in jurisdictions like England, where use rates of over 90 percent are maintained (Mackay, 1985). However, considerable numbers of lives have been saved as a result of existing mandatory use laws. According to NHTSA (National Center for Statistics and Analysis, 1990b), "At the current use level in belt law States (52%), belts would have saved 5,540 lives nationally if all States had belt laws in 1989." Enforcement campaigns for seat belt use laws (encouraged by NHTSA) aim to increase use to 70 percent by 1992.

Some recent studies have confirmed an effect of mandatory seat belt use laws on the patterns of injury of surviving drivers. In Monroe County (Rochester), New York, it was found that hospital admissions of automobile occupants declined 12 percent between the eighteen months prior to the state's belt law and the eighteen months subsequent to the law, while admissions of highway users not covered by the law (motorcyclists, bicyclists, and pedestrians) increased 3 percent (States et al., 1990). The average injury severity score for those admitted was 9 percent lower among automobile occupants, compared with a slight increase for the comparison group. Specifically, major head injuries declined by 18 percent for the occupants compared with a 3.5 percent increase for the controls. Minor head injuries declined by 25 percent, compared with a 10 percent increase among controls. Safety belt use, as determined by either the police report or hospital records, increased from 11 percent to 53 percent. Although some of these differences may lack statistical significance because of small numbers, they are suggestive, and they are confirmed by a study of a sample of admissions to hospital emergency rooms in Suffolk County, New York (Barancik et al., 1988). Admissions as a result of automobile-related injuries decreased, especially in the first trimester under the new law, and fatalities as a proportion of injuries declined considerably, especially among patients with head injuries. A similar study in Charlottesville, Virginia, under a law permitting secondary enforcement only, reported important increases in reported restraint use among occupants of vehicles that had to be towed following crashes. There were also decreases in injuries, especially in circumstances in which theory suggests belts are most likely to be effective (front-seat passengers, frontal crashes), and detailed data indicated that these were obtained by reductions in impacts with windshields and instrument panels (Lestina et al., 1991).

Incentives

It seems possible to increase seat belt use by offering rewards to drivers as well as by threatening them with punishment. Compared with the benefits to the driving population in terms of reduced risks of death and injury, the cost of rewards has been trivial. However, in favorable circumstances their effectiveness in raising seat belt use can be of the same order as that of mandatory use laws, without involving the negatives of punishment-centered policies.

A number of studies of belt-wearing incentive campaigns have been conducted in areas that do not have mandatory use laws. Settings for these campaigns include schools, industrial organizations, and even entire communities. In a typical program, observers monitor parking lots and reward belt users with small, often donated, items such as novelty goods (key chains, credit card wallets), coupons for soft drinks and hamburgers, or tickets for lottery prizes.

In some studies undertaken in North Carolina (Stutts, Hunter, and Campbell, 1984), incentive programs were introduced as phases in campaigns that also contained educational phases. The education programs typically produced small increments in belt wearing, but these were overshadowed by what was achieved with incentives. For example, at Chapel Hill High School, belt wearing rates rose from 20 percent at the baseline to 34 percent in the educational phase, to 53 percent during the incentive program (at one point exceeding 60 percent in response to the promise of funding for a class dance). At the local Blue Cross-Blue Shield office, where the baseline of belt use was less than 10 percent, a four-week incentive program using $5.00 rewards attained use rates of more than 50 percent. A communitywide campaign based on incentives in the Chapel Hill area resulted in more than a 70 percent increase in belt use. Several field studies in southwest Virginia manufacturing sites obtained similar results (Geller and Bigelow, 1984). A study of Dutch army camps (Hagenzieker, 1990) reported that an incentive program offering a reward to the base with the highest belt use rate showed positive findings, of the same magnitude as those of law enforcement strategies.

Although all the studies showed evidence of lower belt use rates once the reward programs terminated, most reported that the last- measured rates were considerably above baseline levels and appeared to be stable. If repeated campaigns prove capable of ratcheting use rates to higher levels, there appears to be considerable value in these programs. As with the punitive approach of mandatory use laws, incentive programs appear to reach populations differentially—for example, white-collar employees appear to change their behavior more than do blue-collar employees—but when these resistant populations are identified it may be possible to create special programs to reach them. Some such success has been reported by Geller (1983).

A principal limitation of incentives programs is the need for a group or, at least, a community base. The suggestion that insurance discounts might serve as general incentives for belt wearing has been rejected by commentators familiar with the situation on two counts: only a small part of the insurance risk could be influenced by this behavior, thus limiting the size of the incentive that could be offered; and experience has found that programs that increase insurance death benefits for belt wearers have not increased the use rate (Williams and Lund, 1988: 52–53). Moreover, it may be difficult in practice to prove belt use in specific collisions.

Passive restraints

Rather than influencing individuals to act to secure protective devices around themselves, it is possible to design protective devices so that no affirmative action by the user is necessary. As noted by Hoffman (1973: 101), "[W]hat technology has uniquely to offer to the solution of complex problems is a kind of option- reducing potential—the possibility of at least removing the decision from the individual (whom we have failed to change time and time again) to the societal level."

Two kinds of technology are relevant here: automatic seat belts and air bags.

The most common passive restraints in contemporary cars are automatic seat belts. Several general types of automatic belt systems have been developed in response to the mandate of Federal Motor Vehicle Safety Standard 208. These are: (1) nonmotorized, detachable, two-point belts (usually with manual lap belts); (2) nonmotorized, detachable, three-point (lap and shoulder) belts; (3) motorized, nondetachable, two-point (shoulder only) belts, with which manual lap belts are provided; (4) motorized, detachable, two-point belts (with manual lap belts). Nonmotorized belts are attached to the door and wrap around the occupant when it closes, whereas motorized ones secure the occupant by gliding in a track around the door when the ignition is turned on.

Observational studies of seat belt use in four metropolitan areas were mounted in 1987 and 1989 by the Insurance Institute for Highway Safety. In the more recent study (Williams et al., 1990) driver shoulder-belt use reached 78 percent in the cars with automatic belts, compared with just 63 percent in cars with manual belts only. (Belt use was 66 percent in cars with both manual belts and air bags, indicating that drivers will not necessarily forego the advantages of seat belts if provided with air bags.) Furthermore, belt use rates differed importantly among the types of automatic devices. The nonmotorized, detachable two-point belts (Type 1) were used by 75 percent, and the nonmotorized, detachable, three-point belts (Type 2) were used by only 66 percent of drivers. The motorized, nondetachable belts (Type 3) had a use rate of 92 percent. The motorized, detachable belts (Type 4) were used by 83 percent of drivers. In brief, drivers sometimes intervened to circumvent the protective devices provided, especially when the technology allowed for detachment and when it was most intrusive and presumably most annoying (Type 2).

The research also found that manual lap belt use was *less* frequent with automatic shoulder belts than when the entire system was manual. The two-point automatic systems yielded more use of shoulder belts but less use of lap belts, apparently compromising some of the effectiveness of the total restraint system. The effect of this loss may be partly compensated by the knee bolsters provided in cars with automatic two-point belt systems.

In sum, evidence finds that automatic seat belt systems result in high levels of protection, clearly exceeding what has been accomplished with manual systems, even when use of the latter is required by law or encouraged with incentives. However, a significant fraction of drivers manage to negate the advantages of these systems by detaching or disabling the shoulder belts and by failing to attach their manual lap belts.

Perhaps the ultimate automatic restraint system is the air bag, which requires no occupant action to be effective. In a frontal or front-angle crash above a given severity, an automatic sensor inflates the bag, providing a yielding surface for the occupant's body. Given its unobtrusiveness, it is difficult to imagine rational vehicle occupants inactivating an air bag system. The protective potential of the device is in theory considerable, though not as great as that of seat belts because its operation and effectiveness are limited to frontal and near-frontal collisions, and to the primary collision rather than to secondary ones that may follow in a complex crash scenario.

The National Highway Traffic Safety Administration (1984) assembled results of four field studies of air bag effectiveness to justify its final ruling on occupant protection in 1984. Air bags alone were estimated likely to reduce occupant fatalities in crashes (regardless of direction) between 20 and 40 percent if used without lap belts. With buckled lap and shoulder belts, savings were estimated between 45 and 55 percent. Although manual lap and shoulder belts were judged capable of nearly the same reductions (40 to 50 percent), this protection would require universal use, a seemingly unattainable goal.

Evans (1988), using his paired-comparison technique, estimated the fatality-preventing effectiveness of air bags alone at 18 percent. His estimate of the effectiveness of lap and shoulder belts was 31 percent. Although Evans's estimates for both devices were lower than those of NHTSA, they concur in finding the belts alone superior to the air bags alone. It should be kept in mind, however, that the effectiveness of unfastened seat belts is zero and that occupants of the vehicles most likely to experience crashes are the most likely to be unbelted.

Clearly, the best that current vehicle technology has to offer for attenuating the link between crashes and injury is a combination of seat belts and air bags. As Williams and Lund (1988: 68) note, "Air bags provide a baseline of protection to those car occupants who do not comply with belt use laws and add to the protection of those who do use belts, particularly by preventing head and face contacts with interior structures in high-speed frontal collisions." As an example of the potential of this technology, Williams and Lund offer the estimate that with a 50 percent belt use rate in America, the lives saved would be approximately doubled, to more than ten thousand annually, with the addition of air bags. The savings due to the air bag would be proportionately greater with lower belt use rates.

Attenuation of the link between crashes and injuries is a major opportunity for lifesaving, and the good news here is that effective technology is rapidly being applied. Seat belts have been standard equipment in cars sold in America for nearly three decades, and either driver air bags or automatic belts have been standard in all cars since the 1990 model year. Many manufacturers currently provide driver-side air bags in their products, and full air-bag protection for front-seat occupants will be provided for vehicles produced by 1993, in compliance with federal law. Numerous lives are now being saved by this technology, and even more will be saved in the future.

The downside of this optimistic picture mainly concerns the time lapse encountered in providing this protection for all vehicles on the road. The new technology has been appearing first on vehicles that in other respects are the safest, that is, large, heavy, luxury cars. Full-size cars have crash-related death rates less than half those of subcompacts, in the absence of air bag and seat belt technology. These vehicles tend to be driven by the safest drivers, who are favored in the distribution of crash forces by the relative weight and other characteristics of their cars. The protection afforded by air bags will come last to younger and poorer people, whose vehicles if new tend to be cheaper, smaller, and lighter and who are disproportionately likely to own older, used cars equipped with the technology of several years ago. These are also the drivers who tend to experience higher than average crash rates and who are least likely to use the manual seat belts in older cars.

The policy implications of these observations are that swift installation of complete occupant protection technology should be encouraged and that manufacturers should be urged through rules or subsidies to make the changes first on models with the highest crash rates. Since retrofitting air bags to older cars appears economically infeasible, turnover of the vehicle fleet should be encouraged, again perhaps with subsidies. In addition, both enforcement of mandatory use laws and, where feasible, belt use incentives systems should be continued.

Addressing the link between injury and death

The final link between drunk driving and the loss of lives is that between injury and death. If ways can be found to treat crash-related injuries so as to prevent them from developing into fatalities, lives will be saved even though the rest of the causal chain remains intact. It appears that the injury-death link, like the others discussed, is characterized by past progress and current opportunity. Unfortunately, much of the research on this topic has been done by medical personnel untrained in scientific research methods. The samples are often small and not representative of larger populations, the comparisons often lack standard tests of statistical significance, and the programs' effects must usually be regarded as approximate.

Interventions addressing this link are especially relevant to deaths caused by drunk driving. Not only are the impaired more likely to experience crashes, but the presence of alcohol is associated with a diminished ability to survive trauma (Evans, 1991). Evans and Frick (1990) estimate that the fatality risk of crash-involved drivers with a BAC of 0.10 percent is roughly double that of drivers with no alcohol in the blood, and that of drivers with a BAC of 0.25 percent is more than tripled. Fell and Hertz (1990), using the FARS data base, have also studied the topic. They report that alcohol increases not only the risk of crash involvement, but also the chance of experiencing more serious injuries and dying in consequence. The drinker's body is less able than that of the nondrinker to withstand trauma stresses, and death comes more quickly. Therefore, techniques for medically addressing injury are disproportionately likely to be beneficial in crashes where alcohol is present.

The success of medical treatment in coping with trauma is vitally a function of the swiftness with which the treatment is made available. A large proportion of crash-related deaths occur before the victim arrives at a hospital, and according to studies based on autopsy reports, many who die might have survived had they received more prompt care (Bota and Cox, 1986; Frey, Huelke, and Gikas, 1969). The problem of delayed care is most serious in sparsely settled states, in rural areas, late at night, and on Interstates (Brodsky, 1990). A seriously injured person can go into irremediable shock in fifteen to twenty minutes, yet delays of a half-hour and more are experienced in nearly one out of five rural fatal accidents.

Delay in providing emergency medical care has begun to be addressed in many places through the establishment of helicopter rescue services, which are capable of bringing injured persons from isolated sites to major hospitals far more quickly than had previously been the case. The staff of these services is also likely to be better trained to administer trauma care than previous or typical ambulance service personnel. In a study of one such facility, Baxt and Moody (1983) compared survival rates of patients taken to the same hospital trauma unit by traditional land services and by a model helicopter service. Among the former, fifteen were projected to die on the basis of a statistical index of the seriousness of their injuries; nineteen patients actually died. Among the latter—those transported by the helicopter service—twenty-one were expected to die, but only ten did. Indeed, helicopter-borne patients who died succumbed to more serious injuries than those who died in the ambulance-borne group. However, although the cited studies support the effectiveness of helicopter rescue service, they do not address the costs. A definitive evaluation of helicopter-based rescue service will have to take into account the large cost of establishing and maintaining it.

The skill of emergency personnel is independently related to successful medical intervention. A study of two emergency medical services in Boston, one offering Advanced Life Support services and one the traditional Basic Life Support, found that although there were no differences in the time elapsed in getting patients to the hospital, patients transported by the more skilled team arrived in better shape and had a higher probability of surviving (Jacobs et al., 1984). This was especially true for persons with moderate injuries, as opposed to those seriously injured.

A similar conclusion was reached in analysis of a natural experiment concerning people jumping from a bridge in Seattle, Washington (Fortner et al., 1983). The survival rate tripled following establishment of the city's Medic 1 program for training the Fire Department staff responsible for transporting injured persons.

Improvement in the quality of care available at hospitals also appears to help prevent deaths from injuries suffered in crashes. A study of two California locations found that trauma victims brought to a central specialized trauma center in San Francisco County were more likely to survive than victims brought to the nearest hospital emergency room in Orange County, even though on average the latter received care more quickly (West, Trunkey, and Lim, 1979). On the basis of a review of records, numerous possible errors in the medical management of the Orange County cases were indicated. The researchers concluded,

Our data suggest that the San Francisco County system, which includes a trauma center, works quite well, while the Orange County system, which lacks a trauma center, does not. Of 92 consecutive deaths in San Francisco County, only one was judged potentially preventable. On the other hand, we believe that a substantial fraction, perhaps as much as 73% of the non-CNS [central nervous system]-related deaths and 28% of the CNS-related deaths in Orange County, could have been prevented with vigorous resuscitation and aggressive surgical intervention. [458]

A correlational study among Florida counties found that the traffic death rate was related both to the presence of an advanced life support system and to the presence of higher-quality hospital facilities (Alexander et al., 1984). This relation was true even though no hospital in the state provided trauma care in compliance with standards enunciated by the American College of Surgeons.

A major limitation of emergency medical services in addressing serious highway crashes has been that the services have tended to cluster in urban areas, whereas fatal crashes are largely rural. Extensions of these services into rural areas, as in the case of the helicopter services mentioned above, may prove disproportionately beneficial in reducing crash-related fatalities.

Another limitation of emergency medical services is that they must be summoned before being able to respond to an emergency, and this notification process is generally beyond the control of medical agencies. The need for services must be observed and reported by someone. Citizen reports are usually to police, who then alert the provider of emergency medical services. Only at that point can response, such as sending an ambulance, begin. Although there is evidence that response delays in highway crashes have been reduced over the last several years, communication and notification delays continue to contribute significantly to the failure of services to reach the needy in time to be of assistance (Brodsky, 1990). This problem may be addressed in part by technology—for example, providing emergency telephones on heavily traveled roads such as Interstates—and in part by policy—for example, immediately dispatching an ambulance on receipt of word of a serious crash, regardless of whether injuries are mentioned.

The materials in this chapter are based on the assumption that drunk driving, while it can be reduced by policies discussed in previous chapters, is unlikely to be eliminated. If impaired drivers continue to be present on the roads, the policies discussed here can reduce the death rate from drivers who continue to drive while impaired and thus contribute to the lowering of the social toll associated with drunk driving. They can also be effective in saving lives threatened by causes other than drunk driving.

The policies are addressed to weakening the links between impairment, error, crashes, injuries, and death. Impairment need not lead to error if, for example, the driving task is simplified through a reduction of the conflict of streams of traffic. Error need not lead to crashes if, for example, unnecessary obstacles are removed from the roadside. Crashes need not lead to injury if, for example, seat belts are worn and vehicles are equipped with air bags. Injury need not lead to death if, for example, skilled medical care is made available promptly. Although these policies may not operate perfectly, they are proven to be effective and offer promise for saving lives in the future.

Paradigms and Policies

This book aims to broaden the understanding of impaired driving and the conception of the drunk driving problem on the part of citizens and political leaders in America. It hopes to supplement the prevailing view, which I term the dominant paradigm, according to which drunk driving is viewed as fundamentally deviant, with a broader one, the challenging paradigm, which views drunk driving as a predictable consequence of existing social institutions. Adherence to the challenging paradigm does not require abandonment of the view that drunk driving is a crime, but it requires that such an understanding be supplemented through an acknowledgment of causal, legal, and moral complexities. The broader understanding of the drunk driving problem in the challenging paradigm leads to a broader program of countermeasures focused on the ultimate goal, that of saving lives.

Paradigms of drunk driving

Paradigms are intellectual models of the world around us. All paradigms are simplifications. The serve as aids to understanding, not literal representations of reality. The paradigms according to which social problems are understood have implications for policy, and criticism of policy often involves questioning the underlying paradigm. For example, the proposal to reduce the numbers of missing children by increasing the penalty for kidnapping assumes that the problem is one of abduction by strangers, while opponents rely on the different understanding that missing children often are runaways who usually return home on their own, or who, if

7

younger, often have been taken from legal custody by a noncustodial parent (Best, 1989; Finkelhor, Hotaling, and Sedlak, 1990).

Elements of the models of drunk driving which I refer to as dominant and challenging paradigms have both been present in discussions of traffic safety for several decades. The dominant paradigm is not obsolete and the challenging one is not unprecedented. The debate over drunk driving policy often includes elements of both paradigms. However, their relative prominence in the discussion is shifting, with an increasing policy role for measures related to the challenging paradigm. The paradigms differ in their understandings of the nature, the size, and the causes of the problem, and in their implications for policy. I present here a summary of their contents.

The dominant paradigm

The dominant paradigm by which drunk driving is understood focuses on a blameworthy driver. This driver is dangerous, and the danger is realized in the form of death and injury. The villain is the "killer drunk," typified by Clarence Busch, the driver who inadvertently stimulated the founding of Mothers Against Drunk Driving when he ran over Candy Lightner's thirteen-year-old daughter, Cari. The killer drunk not only has an extraordinarily high BAC; he is also extremely and obviously impaired in his behavior. Moreover, this is not his first brush with danger on the highway—he has a long history of prior crashes and of previous contacts with an ineffective legal system. Clarence Busch had three prior drunk driving convictions on his record the day he killed Cari Lightner, yet he had spent a mere forty-eight hours in jail. His culpability was underlined by his failure to stop after he hit the child (Steinbock, 1985).

Rather than conceiving of danger as being inherent in all drinking and driving, the dominant paradigm understands there to be a safe drinking level for driving, differentiated from drunk driving. The social drinker who has a couple of beers before driving is safe. He knows and respects his limits. His drinking and driving is therefore responsible. However, beyond some implicit limit lies dangerous and irresponsible drunk driving, qualitatively different from the safe and responsible. The distinction is fundamental, dividing sheep from goats, the massive numbers of ordinary, conventional, good people who drink socially from a small proportion of bad, blameworthy deviants who drink and drive irresponsibly.

The dominant paradigm also presumes the presence of an innocent victim in alcohol-related crashes. The victim is viewed as a nondrinker and likely a nondriver such as a pedestrian or bicyclist, whose use of the road is violently interrupted by the impact of the villain's vehicle. Cari Lightner, whose innocence was underscored by her youth, typifies this victim especially well.

Those who hold to the dominant paradigm understand the behavior described by this typification to be the cause of something like half of the more than forty thousand crash-related fatalities occurring in the United States every year. Data indicating that in about half of all fatal crashes some individual has been found with alcohol in his blood are offered in support of this belief.

Because the dominant paradigm sees drunk driving as attributable to a small, culpable minority of irresponsible individuals, it views the problem as a matter that can and ought to be dealt with by the criminal law. The punishment administered is not only seen as being justified, but is also believed to be capable of reducing further criminality by confirming the threat of swift, sure, and severe punishment for the offenders.

This paradigm reigns in current public understanding and public policy despite its fundamental flaws. Briefly, the dominant paradigm combines an image of the size of the drunk driving problem based on the total numbers of alcohol-involved fatal crashes with an understanding of the nature of the problem based on a small and unrepresentative sample of these crashes. If the problem is the slaughter of innocents by killer drunks, then it is much smaller than the paradigm suggests, whereas if drunk driving is the most widespread crime and among the leading causes of death in America then the distinction between victims and villains, and the attribution of gross culpability to the latter, must fall.

The dominant paradigm experiences difficulty in accounting for several kinds of empirical data. Among these are the following:

First, although it is true that the bulk of serious alcohol-related crashes involve drivers with high BACs, these drivers seldom fit the image of the killer drunk. Their impairment, while dangerous, is often hard to detect in their behavior, even when they are examined by experts, including police and physicians. Most of them lack prior convictions for drunk driving. Beyond this, no qualitative distinctions can be found in practice between impaired and unimpaired drivers who drink. An increase in crash risk appears to begin with the lowest detectable BACs, and it rises progressively and geometrically, smoothly and without inflection, as BACs rise. At BACs produced by normative, or "social," drinking, the risk of fatal crashes doubles and quadruples, resulting in large numbers of fatal crashes in which alcohol impairment is involved and even causal, though not illegal. Of course, much higher multiples of crash risk occur for heavier drinkers.

Second, the typical victim of drunk driving is the drunk driver himself. More than half of all people killed in alcohol-involved crashes are drivers with BACs of 0.10% and higher. Another fifth are passengers in the drunk driver's car, whose BACs are generally similar to that of the driver. Another tenth are alcohol-impaired pedestrians and cyclists who are struck by motor vehicles. Although victims resembling Cari Lightner are altogether too frequent, they are a small and atypical fraction of people killed in alcohol-involved crashes. If lives lost to drunk driving are to be saved, most of them will pertain to drunk drivers. Only a small minority of those killed are innocent victims in the sense of having been unimpaired by alcohol at the time of the crash and presumably without responsibility for its occurrence (National Highway Traffic Safety Administration, 1991).

Third, drunk driving is not as deviant as is suggested in the dominant paradigm. Drinking to the point at which the drinker is significantly impaired in driving a vehicle is socially accepted in America, and drinking to BACs that yield extraordinary multiples of serious crash risk is tolerated and even expected in particular social strata (Wechsler and Isaac, 1991). Although heavy drinkers are dangerous on the highway, it is not necessary to view them as abnormal or pathological; they may be drinking in accord with the norms of heavy-drinking social subgroups.

Large proportions of drinkers admit in interviews to having driven after drinking in the recent past and to expectations that they will drink and drive in the future. The suggestion in the dominant paradigm that only small numbers of people drive while impaired fails to appreciate both the widespread nature of impaired driving and the fact that its roots lie in social institutions.

The challenging paradigm

In the challenging paradigm, drunk driving is an understandable, predictable product of social institutions, reinforced by interests vested in their maintenance. The institutions in question are recreation and transportation, which assume drinking and driving, respectively. The intersection of these institutions, which is predictable and unremarkable, produces drunk driving as a consequence. There is nothing inherently wrong about this structuring of society, but it does produce unintended and undesired results along with those we value positively.

The challenging paradigm recognizes that heavy drinkers are at the core of the problem but that they are not the only ones in that position. It does not accept a fundamental distinction between the safe and the dangerous, between conventional sheep and deviant goats. Moderate or social drinkers contribute to the drunk driving problem, and there are no obvious lines to draw between moderate and heavy drinkers. Using the language of alcoholic beverage commercials, there are no limits to know. No significant amount of drinking can be termed responsible for someone who intends to drive. What is more, the norms that lead to much heavy drinking, though damaging, are not necessarily perverse or deviant. Rather, they are often variant, different in degree rather than in kind from general norms regarding drinking in America.

The challenging paradigm also embraces the public health criterion that reduced deaths and injuries are the bottom line for developing policy. Righting the moral balance of the world, or securing justice, is not the central concern in this paradigm. Deterrence-based policies are accepted in the challenging paradigm to the degree that they produce empirical effectiveness rather than for their retributive appropriateness. Policies based on increasing the severity of punishment for drunk drivers beyond that prevailing today have seldom been found effective and are regarded with skepticism in the challenging paradigm, whereas those emphasizing certainty and swiftness of punishment are regarded as promising.

The challenging paradigm draws on the disillusionment of social scientists with the results of criminal punishment, with respect not only to drunk driving but also to more conventionally imaged crimes such as robbery and assault. In general, the various punishments experienced by criminals cannot be shown to have changed these offenders and to have reduced their subsequent law violations. "[F]rom the point of view of individual prevention, the best result is obtained by desisting from all coercive measures" (Mäkelä, 1978: 328). Moreover, for many crimes, including serious drunk driving, most damage is inflicted by people who have not previously been caught and who therefore could not have experienced criminal sanctions. Even if sanctions were effective in changing known law violators, they could have little direct effect on overall crime. Of course, criminal punishment of offenders may, through the general deterrence mechanism, affect the behavior of people not directly punished. This potential has been demonstrated on occasions, both for drunk driving and for street crimes, when a deterrent threat's swiftness and certainty were strengthened by measures like well- publicized enforcement campaigns. However, perhaps in part because actual enforcement has often been halfhearted or limited in time, these accomplishments most commonly have been temporary, with matters eventually reverting to the former status quo (Ross and LaFree, 1986).

As I have argued throughout this book, there is growing evidence that policies other than those based in criminal justice, operating through mechanisms other than deterrence, can be effective in reducing problematic behavior. Many of the successful interventions have in common a basis in a sociological understanding of the causes of the behavior in question. They are directed to reducing the situational inducements and incentives to engage in the prohibited behavior, rather than to increasing the punishment threatened for engaging in it.

The challenging paradigm adds policies relevant to alcohol consumption to the arsenal of social weapons used to fight drunk driving. These are expected to operate without any necessary relationship to negligence and culpability. The dangers of using alcohol, including drunk driving, are approached through increasing the price, reducing the availability, and changing the marketing of alcoholic beverages. The promise of these countermeasures is illustrated by the success of the national minimum drinking age laws. However, most potentially effective alcohol-based policies are unlikely to be simple; mere reduction in total consumption may not be the most efficient approach to reducing all alcohol-related problems.

The challenging paradigm includes transportation policy among countermeasures to drunk driving. Like alcohol policy, it is unconcerned with negligence and culpability. Because of society's thorough commitment to automobiles, transportation measures are harder to apply than measures based in alcohol policy, yet they have both short-run and long-run promise for reducing drunk driving. For example, it is possible that the success of minimum drinking age laws in alcohol policy can be paralleled in transportation policy by placing curfews on young people's driving during drinking hours. Inducing people who plan to drink to use means of transportation other than the private car, by such means as subsidies, is also an appealing possibility.

The challenging paradigm further suggests the utility of measures that affect the links between impairment, error, crashes, injuries, and deaths in reducing deaths caused by impairment even though impaired persons continue to drive. Since most of the lives threatened by impaired driving—and thus potentially saved by effective countermeasures—are those of the impaired themselves, these measures are not very attractive by dominant paradigm criteria, which emphasize the impaired drivers' responsibility for their own predicaments. However, they may be among the most important by the standards of the challenging paradigm, which stresses cost-effective savings of lives without regard to issues of personal responsibility.

The politics of drunk driving

Why should drunk driving, or traffic safety more generally, be a political matter, when the issues can be seen as technical and scientific ones? The propriety of involving politicians and the public in these matters has been strongly (and colorfully) challenged by Frank Haight (1983):

The third component of [a traffic-safety] strategy is the gradual disengagement of road safety from public concern and from direct political interference. As Anatol Rapoport . . . says "While there may be no better way to conduct politics than by formal majority-determined elections, referenda, etc., it is not justifiable to extend these decision rules to questions related to public health, public safety, etc." In general the influence of the public, whether directly or through political institutions, has been pernicious to traffic safety. It comes and goes, filling in the troughs between peaks of more exciting events; it seizes on issues without concern for the relevance or tractability of the problems; it proposes "solutions" which are at best naive and at worst absurd, and above all it demands action even where action may be only a waste of money. At a recent large meeting devoted to drunk driving, a prominent speaker put the issue very well. He said, "The American people have refused to say that any problem is insolvable", and the meeting went on to demand

173

immediate implementation of all those countermeasures which so conspicuously failed during the 1970s. [8]

Although it is hard to challenge Haight's characterization of the outcome of the political process in the area of traffic safety, his proposed solution of entrusting the issue to low-profile agencies with legitimacy based on demonstrated accomplishments seems wishful and unrealistic. Indeed, the example he subsequently offers of the Food and Drug Administration is unconvincing in light of the political controversy generated by its drug-approval procedures in the age of AIDS. His viewpoint neglects the fact that the recognition of any condition as a social problem is a political matter. Indeed, the designation of the problem as something to be handled by scientific experts is fundamentally political. It is not helpful for underdogs in the political game to pick up their chips, denounce the rules— "Road safety is driven by political motives and fueled by ignorance" (Hauer, 1990)—and look elsewhere, when the political game is the only game in town. Even the experts are forced to play it, often as mere adjutants to parties with less sophistication but greater involvement and determination (Ross, 1987b; Gordis, 1991).

Political bases of the paradigms

Intellectually, both dominant and challenging paradigms have their origin in the literature of traffic safety, which as an interdisciplinary field embodies the perspectives of disciplines ranging from engineering to psychology. This literature has been produced by technicians and experts, not by the uninformed public. Traditionally, there has been general agreement among traffic safety specialists that "accidents" or "crashes" represent failures of a system, the major components of which are the vehicle, the highway, and the driver. However, the field has split along lines that reflect the different views I have summarized in the paradigms. Participants who have an engineering background have tended to stress vehicle and highway failures as the principal areas of breakdown, whereas those grounded in psychology and similar perspectives have generally emphasized the responsibility of the individual driver to compensate for defects in the vehicle and the highway and have viewed system breakdowns primarily as driver failures.

The epithet identified with this latter view is "The nut that holds the wheel," pointing to a classic villain devised and marketed to the public over many decades by the traffic safety division of the National Safety Council. The similarity of this character to the killer drunk of the dominant drunk driving paradigm is evident, and indeed much safety literature researching the causes of driver failure has identified its causes in alcohol impairment. Perhaps the landmark in this tradition was an early report, *Alcohol and Highway Safety* (U.S. Congress, 1968), from the National Highway Safety Bureau, forerunner of the National Highway Traffic Safety Administration (NHTSA). This document pointed to alcohol as a major source of fatal crashes and to the crucial role of heavy drinkers. Furthermore, it accepted the ideas of guilt and innocence in the causation of crashes:

The use of alcohol by drivers and pedestrians leads to some 25,000 deaths and a total of at least 800,000 crashes in the United States each year. Especially tragic is the fact that much of the loss in life, limb, and property damage involves completely innocent parties. ... Alcoholics and other problem drinkers, who constitute but a small minority of the general population, account for a very large part of the overall problem. [1]

This view of the drunk driving problem is fully consistent with the dominant paradigm, a matter remarkable because the principal author of the report, Dr. William Haddon, Jr.—the first administrator of the federal highway safety agency—was strongly associated with such challenging paradigm policies as mandating automatic restraints in vehicles to prevent injuries in crashes.

The other tradition in safety thinking rejects the idea of changing the nut, substituting the goal of, in Haddon's (1970) words, "preventing the escape of tigers." It has been more influential in the area of industrial safety than in traffic safety. While people on the automobile side at the National Safety Council were designing training and propaganda programs to improve drivers, those on the industrial safety side were devising guards to prevent fingers from being mutilated by machinery.

Both paradigms were embodied in the activities of the federal traffic safety agency from its founding in 1966. Although concern with vehicle construction and the setting of standards struck most observers as the central theme of the American approach to traffic safety (Irwin, 1985), the sequel to *Alcohol and Highway Safety* was a series of programs across the nation that stressed the criminal justice approach. Alcohol Safety Action Programs were instituted in thirty-five communities in the United States in the early 1970s. Funded with $88 million in federal subsidies and at least that much in additional public and private funds, more than half of the money went to law enforcement (McCarthy, 1990). Further, between 1967 and 1985 nearly $2 billion was allocated by NHTSA to supporting local community traffic safety, and close to half of this went to police traffic services and "alcohol countermeasures" related to the dominant paradigm.

Supporters of the dominant paradigm

The views and policies associated with the dominant paradigm have understandably been popular with people who have directly or indirectly, through friends and relatives, experienced harm in the course of alcohol-related crashes. Many of these have been mobilized in a citizens' or victims' social movement that includes organizations like MADD, founded by Candy Lightner and others in 1980, and Remove Intoxicated Drivers (RID), founded by Doris Aiken in 1978. The movement's basic, though not exclusive, commitment to the dominant paradigm has been documented in several studies (Weed, 1985; McCarthy, Wolfson, and Harvey, 1987; Ungerleider and Bloch, 1988).

For example, MADD's tenth-anniversary program statement (1990) declared,

> Mothers Against Drunk Driving believes that driving impaired by alcohol or other drugs is a crime, and the crashes which result are not accidents.
>
> Virtually every state's laws acknowledge impaired driving as a crime, and the seriousness of the consequences that can result make punitive sanctions appropriate and imperative.
>
> Such sanctions help to prevent repeat offenses as well as to raise public awareness of enforcement efforts. . . . While education and rehabilitation have a role in a comprehensive approach, they are no substitute for firm, effective, sanctions. [9]

The national leadership appears to speak for the local chapters as well in this regard. Ungerleider and Bloch, surveying 212 MADD chapters nationwide, found that "an overwhelming majority (90%) of chapter leaders reported strong legal penalties to be the most effective countermeasure. Strict enforcement of laws was the next most important measure" (1988, 194). They noted an apparent shift from the results of Weed's (1985) earlier survey, which reported that 85 percent of the leadership believed public awareness of drunk driving to be the most important countermeasure and suggested that MADD's orientation was shifting from a position that involved a general interest in prevention to one exclusively centered on criminal justice. (To this observer, the difference was probably a matter of the wording of the questions rather than a change in the views of MADD's leadership.)

The origins of this view in tragic personal experiences, recounted in nearly every issue of MADD's newsletters, is comprehensible. MADD is, after all, an organization of victims devoted to securing justice and recompense for those harmed as well as to preventing future drunk driving. What requires explanation is how relatively small interest groups like MADD and RID have been able to determine the public conception of a problem and to influence adoption of the countermeasures deemed effective by this view. The fact is that although MADD can legitimately claim large numbers of contributors and supporters—it raised $43.5 million from contributions in 1989—the number of active members in all organizations pertaining to the citizens' movement against drunk driving is surprisingly small. In 1985, when it reached perhaps the height of its political influence, MADD had some 377 chapters nationally (McCarthy, 1990). RID, which though older seems destined perpetually to play Avis to MADD's Hertz, had approximately 70 chapters. Including independent groups, the total numbers of chapters of anti-drunk driving citizens' organizations amounted to fewer than 500. Since the average chapter counted about 35 members, one can conclude that the total active membership of the movement was less than 20,000 nationwide. This figure may be compared, for example, with the 2.7 million members of the National Rifle Association or the more than 32 million members of the American Association of Retired Persons.

Much of the effectiveness of the citizens' movement is due to its alliance with the traffic safety establishment. State and federal officials have found the movement useful for demonstrating popular support for statutes and other measures proposed by the safety agencies, while the programs endorsed by the movement have been rendered rational and politically sophisticated in the process. The NHTSA has explicitly recognized the value of this constituency and has taken steps to enlarge and strengthen it:

> In 1979 the agency published and widely distributed a guide describing in great detail how to start a citizens' group opposing drinking and driving. The effectiveness of this guide as an organizational template for local groups is evidenced by the correspondence between its suggestions and the basic structure of the local citizens' groups we have studied. . . . The availability of this organizational technology no doubt facilitated the growth of local groups around the country. [McCarthy et al., 1988: 74]

The NHTSA continues to nurture movement organizations through small grants, sponsorship of national conferences, the provision of expertise in the preparation of programs, and other means.

The movement also appears powerful because of its alliance with other interests rooted in the dominant paradigm. These were well represented in the membership of the Presidential Commission on Drunk Driving (1983) and in that of its successor organization, the National Commission Against Drunk Driving. Among these interests are law enforcement, which uses the dominant paradigm to argue for additions to personnel and equipment; safety educators, trainers, and alcohol therapists, whose programs obtain considerable enrollment among drunk drivers who otherwise face jail and license revocation (Langton, 1991: 174–75); and a new class of entrepreneurs providing products such as server intervention training, breath-alcohol interlocks, and prevention programs (e.g., Students Against Driving Drunk, or SADD). The nature of the interests involved is clear, and their adoption of the dominant paradigm of drunk driving is understandable.

Perhaps less obvious is the compatibility of anti-drunk-driving policies that assume the dominant paradigm with the interests of both the alcoholic beverage industry and such alcohol industry clients as the media. This compatibility is witnessed by the fact that the industries have at one time or another been important contributors to citizens' movement groups (with the notable exception of RID), and they have been the principal sponsors of related programs such as the high–school based SADD and the college–based BACCHUS (Montague, 1989). The alcohol industry cannot and does not deny the existence of alcohol problems. It accepts an obligation to contribute to the reduction of these problems. However, it defines the problems as based on misuse of the product and views them as limited to a small minority of drinkers (Langton, 1991; Ross, 1986). This perception fits well with the dominant paradigm, in which killer drunks are easily seen as alcohol abusers who form a small proportion of all drinkers. It fits less well with the challenging paradigm, which sees some risk of alcohol-related death and injury at all levels of alcohol consumption and no exemption of normative or acceptable drinking from contributing to deaths in alcohol-related crashes.

Both the alcohol and broadcasting industries have supported the National Commission Against Drunk Driving while working to undermine the Surgeon General's Workshop on Drunk Driving, which launched the challenging paradigm into the national discourse, and the organization that evolved from it, the National Coalition to Prevent Impaired Driving.

This is not to say that the alcohol industry and related industries were ever the major source of funding for any citizens' movement organizations or, more important, that their support necessarily affected the program or philosophy of particular groups. Rather, the affinity between the viewpoints of most of the groups and those of the industries led to joint support of policies based on the dominant paradigm and increased the political effectiveness of the citizens' movements.

The influence of the citizens' movement has also been magnified by media interest. Victims have traditionally been quite attractive to the media. According to Gans's (1979) content analysis of news media, between 20 and 25 percent of magazine columns that deal with unknowns, or ordinary people (as opposed to knowns—government officials and celebrities), are concerned with victims of natural or social disorders. They were the subject of 33 percent of television news stories dealing with unknowns. If stories about "alleged and actual violators of the laws and mores" are added to victim stories, the total proportion of stories centering on subjects comparable to drunk driving amounts to about 40 percent of those dealing with ordinary people in both types of media. Stories that relate tragic events involving victims and villains are clearly very attractive to the media.

After Clarence Busch, in a state of alcoholic impairment, ran over Cari Lightner, Candy Lightner had a tragic story to tell. She told it very well, eventually even in a film made for national television. Much the same can be said for hundreds of other people whose lives have been devastated by the consequences of crashes involving alcohol in communities across the country. Although media reporting of stories related to drunk driving peaked in 1983 and has declined in subsequent years, it persists at a high level compared to prior decades (McCarthy et al., 1988).

Finally, drunk driving policies based on the dominant paradigm fit easily into a political environment in which conservative political and social philosophies reign. In the 1980s, ideas reflecting conservative conceptions of society became more acceptable than in previous decades: social problems stem from individual deviant acts; individual deviants deserve full blame for social problems; and the infliction of punishment is a legitimate and effective means of dealing with and reducing deviance. This fit is the basis of a sociological analysis of MADD by Craig Reinarman (1988). Although his characterization of the organization may strike one as oversimplified and somewhat dated, it is appropriate as an analysis of the appeal of dominant paradigm thinking at a given time in history:

> Each of these major facets of MADD's orientation—its individualist focus, its systematic inattention to structural/corporate sources of problems, and its narrow retributive prescriptions—is in ideological harmony with and gains legitimacy from the policies and the rhetoric of Reagan and the New Right. There is also some preliminary evidence on the social base of the movement that supports such an interpretation. . . . [T]he rate of MADD Chapter formation across states and regions of the United States is strongly correlated with standard survey measures of politico-religious conservatism. [106]

As Reinarman cautions, this congruence should not be construed as causal in any rigorous sense, but it does suggest another reason why a citizens' movement against drunk driving flourished in the 1980s while the role of alcohol in highway fatalities was declining.

Supporters of the challenging paradigm

The challenging paradigm is politically centered in the public health profession and in organizations that belong to the consumers' movement. It is popular among civil libertarians, who are concerned about the expansion of police activity produced by the need to enforce drunk driving laws (Jacobs, 1989), and among attorneys who, in defending accused drivers, have found themselves being accused as accessories after the fact in drunk driving crimes. The challenging paradigm is also supported by important segments of groups that support the dominant paradigm—both traffic safety agencies and citizens' movement organizations—but, unlike the dominant one, it evokes considerable political opposition as well.

The challenging paradigm has been prominent in the general approach to alcohol problems taken by public health officials. The Surgeon General's Workshop, held in Washington, D.C., in December 1988, gave these officials a central place in the formal consideration of drunk driving. (Its final report was issued in May 1989.) The workshop was called largely in response to congressional resolutions obtained by citizen activists associated with the dominant paradigm of drunk driving. Planning for the workshop, however, included persons with public health backgrounds, namely, representatives of the U.S. Public Health Service. The workshop thus yielded sessions, reports, and eventually recommendations in areas new to the politics of drunk driving. Important among these were the control of alcohol consumption through pricing and constraints on availability, advertising, and marketing, the control of driving through transportation policy, and the control of injuries notwithstanding drunk driving (Office of the Surgeon General, 1989).

The Surgeon General's Workshop did not reject the dominant paradigm, but rather joined it to the challenging one to a degree unprecedented in previous official reports on drunk driving. Drunk driving was seen not as an isolated phenomenon but as part of two larger social problems, which might be called the alcohol problem and the traffic safety problem. The workshop found that, although deterrent approaches might be useful in dealing with the intersection of these larger problems, their totality would be more successfully addressed by broader measures, operating through market and regulatory mechanisms in addition to those of criminal justice.

If the political times were propitious for the ascendancy of the dominant paradigm, new political realities may prove to have been important in the rise of the challenging paradigm. The Surgeon General's Workshop was held in the last days of the Reagan administration, and a new administration was in place at the time the report was issued. It can be argued that experience had demonstrated some limitations of the conservative approach to social problems not far removed from drunk driving—for example, in the war on drugs. Moreover, although the 1980s saw a decline in the extent of drunk driving, it appears that much of the success not attributable to such extraneous changes as economic and demographic shifts could be ascribed to challenging paradigm policies like the national minimum drinking age. In all events, the numbers of alcohol-related fatalities remained too high to justify complacency with the achievements of the decade.

The organizations representing the citizens' movement against drunk driving, while continuing to support deterrence as a central goal, increasingly appear willing to lend their support to broader policies. RID, for exan ple, has always demanded controls on alcohol advertising, and MADD in 1990 endorsed alcohol taxes, if undertaken to fund other drunk driving programs, and controls on advertising, if directed at young people. RID has made common cause with a variety of consumer and public health organizations by joining the National Coalition to Prevent Impaired Driving (NCPID), an organization emanating from the Surgeon General's Workshop. The NCPID requires members to support the workshop's ten key summary recommendations, including those to increase alcohol taxes and to regulate marketing of alcoholic beverages. Although the national leadership of MADD has declined to endorse the challenging paradigm to the extent of joining NCPID, the surgeon general's recommendations appear to be popular among many of the movement's rank and file.

The momentum of the challenging paradigm appears to be slowed mainly by the fact that some of its policies meet opposition from powerful vested interests. Producers and sellers of alcoholic beverages are scarcely indifferent to the surgeon general's proposals regarding taxation and regulation. Those industries dependent on alcohol promotion—most notably the media, but also amateur and professional sports teams and even colleges and universities—are conflicted.

The National Association of Broadcasters (NAB) first accepted an invitation to the Surgeon General's Workshop on Drunk Driving but later declined because of reservations about balance among the participants in the expert panel on advertising and marketing of alcohol. Other groups closely associated with the alcoholic beverage industry also refused invitations to participate in the workshop. Concern about possible recommendations in the area of taxation and marketing was also expressed in a lawsuit filed by the National Association of Beer Wholesalers (with an amicus brief from the NAB) against the surgeon general on the eve of the workshop. The association sought to prevent the convening of the workshop, even though 120 invited participants were already in Washington and ready to proceed. The suit was brought about by Surgeon General C. Everett Koop's refusal to yield to less formal pressures. Numerous expressions of concern were received by his staff from the affected industries and from Capitol Hill. These included a letter from the NAB to Koop that made a number of charges in what was perceived as an offensive manner. Industry pressure may have been responsible for the failure of several important officials, including the secretary of transportation, the administrator of NHTSA, and the director of the National Commission Against Drunk Driving, to attend as expected. Moreover, although the workshop was convened in the nation's capital, a quintessential media center, neither the workshop nor the lawsuit was mentioned in local or national media at the time. This was all the more remarkable because of the involvement of Koop, a flamboyant, well-known government official, and the timeliness of the topic: the workshop took place just before the Christmas and New Year holidays, when drunk driving is usually a matter of considerable media interest.

Although the Surgeon General's Workshop produced numerous recommendations based on the challenging paradigm, it would be inaccurate to say that the paradigm has yet displaced the dominant one at the forefront of drunk driving policy today. The NHTSA's (1990) plan for the decade of the 1990s, for example, is firmly anchored in deterrence, and the NCPID appears to be having difficulties in obtaining financial support and exerting political influence. There are signs, however, that the situation may be changing. The medical community has employed its prestigious professionals as players in what was formerly a low-status game. The success of public health interests in enacting challenging-paradigm laws and achieving results in the area of smoking prevention cannot be regarded with equanimity by those interested in equanimity by those interested in maintaining current levels of alcohol consumption. Furthermore, the cheapest and most obvious dominant-paradigm policies have already been widely adopted. Improvement the criminal justice system would seem to depend on the adoption of measures that increase the swiftness and certainty of punishment, rather than its severity, and most of these are likely to be expensive. It is possible that they will fail to be supported by a tax-resistant public once their costs become evident. The potential exhaustion of the ability of deterrence-based laws to affect drunk driving with prevailing and foreseeable amounts of resources may be on the horizon. If so, further of resources may be on the horizon. If so, further progress in reducing drunk driving will require other kinds of policies.

Perhaps the greatest contribution of the citizens' movement to controlling drunk driving has been its message that alcohol-related deaths are not inevitable and that we can seek political means to reduce them. If the deterrence-centered measures associated with the movement's commitment to the dominant paradigm have by now yielded most of what they can with the resources available, it is possible that the energy and devotion of movement members can be recruited in support of challenging-paradigm policies that promise to bring further accomplishments. The steps already taken in that direction by MADD and RID suggest that this is not merely wishful thinking.

A program for reducing drunk driving

In this book I have criticized current drunk driving policy in America as being based on a partial understanding of the problem and therefore as yielding less than optimal results. This does not mean that I regard all current policy as misguided or that I counsel complacency and fatalism in the matter of drunk driving. Much of what we are doing is sensible; it appears to be having effects, reducing deaths from what they might have been in the absence of such policy. A better understanding of the problem, however, can yield prescriptions for improved conception and implementation of policy, policy capable of saving further lives. I have noted such opportunities throughout the book.

In the concluding pages, I wish to recapitulate some of these recommendations. They are of two kinds. On the one hand are existing policies that have been proven effective by competent evaluations. On the other are those that are promising but have not been implemented and those that have been implemented but not evaluated. Policies in the first category ought to be retained and given resources in proportion to their effectiveness. Even policies with demonstrated effectiveness, however, may be improved by modifications and variations. For example, if enforcement of deterrence-based laws is found to save lives, policy makers should try to determine the optimal level of enforcement, the best techniques, and where and when they should be applied. If raising alcohol taxes reduces consumption and related problems, they should establish the point at which the benefits diminish because of evasions such as illegal distilling. Policies in both categories can benefit from independent, competent, and repeated scientific evaluation.

Recommendations based in law and criminal justice

One lesson of the deterrence literature that is applicable to drunk driving policy is that increments in severity of threatened punishment beyond levels currently prevailing are most unlikely to achieve substantial and long-lasting decreases in drunk driving. Even if they did, there would be a question of principle concerning the justice of their application. Indeed, the severity of penalties now prescribed is predicated on a misperception of drunk driving that overestimates its risk. Therefore, on a strictly retributive basis, present penalties may be viewed as overly severe for the routine violation. This appears to be the opinion of many judges responsible for deciding drunk driving cases, who find that existing law overstresses punitive objectives (Cowan, Robbins, and Meszaros, 1986). One implication of the prevalence of this belief among participants in the criminal justice system is that they may attempt to avoid imposition of the penalties they view as unfair. There is evidence, for instance, that judges in both Indiana and New Mexico fail to pronounce legislatively mandated jail sentences on many second-offender drunk drivers (Ross and Foley, 1987).

In the area of law and criminal justice the opportunity for further reducing drunk driving lies in increasing the public's perception that swift and sure punishment is meted out for law violations. An obvious example of this opportunity lies in increasing the enforcement of existing laws. When the objective chances of a drunk driver being apprehended lie in the area of 1 in 5,000 miles driven with a BAC of more than 0.10 percent, it is unreasonable to expect the public to view the likelihood of punishment as at all certain. The objective probability of apprehension can be increased in a variety of ways, including the use of sobriety checkpoints at roadblocks, along with more traditional patrol methods such as looking for traffic law violations in the vicinity of taverns. When police crack down on drunk drivers in a well-publicized campaign, the result is often less drunk driving, fewer crashes, and fewer deaths and injuries. The Australian experience suggests that if police activity is maintained, permanent reductions in drunk driving may occur. Moreover, criminological theory leads to the expectation that over time such efforts can permanently affect the public's judgments concerning the acceptability of drinking and driving, thus building constraints against it into social norms and personal values.

Perhaps the main problem in capitalizing on this opportunity is its cost. As Homel says, in reviewing the Australian literature, "the impact of [random breath testing] is pretty much a linear function of the resources devoted to it" (1990: 191–92). Police resources are not cheap, and either the public must be convinced to purchase more of them or resources must be diverted from other pressing crime-control tasks. Even if the monetary expense issue can be avoided, for example, by designating a portion of the income from fines to be returned to the criminal justice system, an increasing of patrols raises questions about the level of police presence Americans will tolerate in their daily lives. If more police are desired and are affordable, the experience of several Australian states, in some ways not too different from our own, demonstrates that in terms of cost-effectiveness—that is, payback in lives saved and injuries reduced—important increments in enforcement are almost certain to be warranted. Furthermore, in Australia, public support for such use of police resources appears to be high, even among drivers stopped for random testing.

The swiftness as well as the certainty of punishment for drunk drivers can be increased through the use of noncriminal sanctioning procedures. The suspension or revocation of licenses by administrative means is practiced by many states, and research supports the potential of this procedure to reduce the recidivism of sanctioned drivers and to deter others. Administrative revocation is a concept rather than a particular statute, and current laws vary in numerous important ways, but all those evaluated demonstrate effectiveness to some degree in reducing drunk driving (Ross, 1991). Most statutes permit the police to take the driver's license at the scene of a failed or refused breath test, replacing it with a temporary permit to drive for a limited number of days. The laws usually provide for prompt administrative hearings of any defenses that might be raised before all driving privileges are lost. Such hearings occur well before the criminal justice system is able to conclude the parallel criminal prosecution. The subsequent suspension or revocation is often about ninety days for initial test failures, with longer periods for subsequent failures and for refusals. There is considerable variation around these general standards, and little is known at present concerning the differences in costs and benefits of the various approaches. As experience with various forms of administrative suspension and revocation laws accumulates, it should be possible to fine-tune the policy to secure maximum deterrence at minimum cost.

A principal problem with administrative suspension or revocation laws is their weak tie to the concurrent criminal prosecution. The dual procedure is complex and confusing, and it leads to potentially conflicting results, such as a finding of good cause for the administrative revocation but a not guilty finding in the criminal case. Although such a discrepancy may not be illogical, given the different standards of proof in the criminal and administrative systems, puzzled drivers found not guilty of drunk driving in court in fact find it hard to comprehend why their licenses are withheld by motor vehicles administrators. Those drivers who claim not to understand the system are most likely to violate suspension or revocation orders (Ross and Gonzales, 1988). To remedy this problem, I recommend that in routine cases the administrative system be substituted in full for the criminal one. Ordinary drunk driving should not be a crime, in the sense of requiring criminal procedures including proof of the offense beyond a reasonable doubt or the imposition of criminal penalties, especially jail. Rather, routine drunk driving should be considered an extremely serious violation of the rules of the road, sanctioned principally by license withdrawal— an action that, although not in theory punitive, is generally experienced as a severe deprivation.

Those wedded to the dominant paradigm of drunk driving might not be able to countenance the suggestion to decriminalize routine offenses, even though replacement of judicial with regulatory procedures could be shown to save lives. Replacement of the criminal by the administrative process, however, would not remove any sanction now applied to drunk drivers except for jail. Given the shortage of jail space in most American communities, this sanction is in fact avoided in routine cases regardless of judicial determination and legislative mandates (Ross and Voas, 1989). Administrators can be empowered to exact fines and fees and to require education and treatment programs in addition to suspending licenses. Exceptional cases of blameworthy behavior—specifically those in which there is evidence of dangerous driving, of death, injury, or other damage, or of an unusually high BAC (and thus potential dangerousness)—would in this proposal remain in the province of the criminal courts. Although in the past the courts have sometimes failed to cope with masses of routine cases, they have seldom dropped the ball when dealing with extreme offenders. I foresee that the consequence of adopting this recommendation would be quicker and more certain punishment for both routine and exceptional offenders, with greater consideration given to the latter by courts no longer overburdened with a flood of routine cases. Were this to occur, theory and experience predict that fewer lives would be lost to drunk driving. If objections on principle to decriminalizing drunk driving can be overcome, and one or more pilot jurisdictions established, a detailed evaluation of an administratively based drunk driving control system would be extremely enlightening.

If the centerpiece of sanctions for drunk drivers is to be license withdrawal, it seems reasonable to look for ways of strengthening this sanction and compelling drivers' compliance to it. Voas's (1988b) suggestions for improving the apprehension rate of unlicensed drivers focus on electronic tagging and sensing devices linked to data bases. Most immediately practicable, and already provided in some states, are special license plates for vehicles owned by persons under suspension or revocation for drunk driving violations (identifying them at least to police as being owned by persons without licenses). The incapacitative effect of license revocation may possibly be improved by the installing of ignition interlocks to prevent vehicles from being driven by someone who has consumed alcohol. For more aggravated defiance of sanctions, such measures as vehicle impoundment and confiscation and house arrest monitored by electronic devices (Schmidt, 1989) might be effective from the viewpoints of special and general deterrence as well as incapacitation. Unfortunately, although these suggestions seem promising (Voas, 1991), there is a dearth of experiences and evaluations concerning them.

Recommendations based in alcohol policy

The most effective recommendation in alcohol policy is to render alcoholic beverages more expensive by increasing excise taxes on them. This can be expected to reduce alcohol consumption by all types of drinkers, heavy as well as light, and thus drunk driving among all types of drinkers. It would, of course, involve renouncing to some degree the positive benefits associated with alcohol consumption. The Surgeon General's Workshop recommended equalizing taxes among beverages for the amount of alcohol contained in them and indexing these for inflation since 1970. Such a tax policy would be expected to give non-alcoholic beverages a price advantage over alcoholic ones, and low-alcohol beverages an advantage over high-alcohol ones. This seems a reasonable, though rather blunt, approach, and modifications should be considered. For example, the relationship of drinking to impaired driving varies with drinking location, and a surtax on drinks consumed in bars might be considered as a partial replacement for a general tax hike. Furthermore, although there is considerable support in research for the general proposition that increasing the price of alcoholic beverages can reduce consumption and related problems, there is disagreement among the studies over the magnitude of the results that can be achieved and relatively little information concerning the benefits possibly foregone because of an increase in the price of drink. More research on these questions is badly needed.

The research literature does not give unqualified support to expectations that manipulating of availability and marketing techniques will reduce drunk driving in the short run, even though such policy accords with intuition and theory. We need to know more about the effectiveness of advertising and its control, especially over the long run. Some alcohol advertising might even be considered useful from a public health viewpoint; for example, advertising might succeed in getting people to substitute low-alcohol for high-alcohol beverages. Similarly, the area of serving practices and server training offers many opportunities for pilot projects and evaluations. The effect of such specific practices as two-for-one promotions and service in undifferentiated containers (e.g., pitchers or kegs of beer) requires more study, extending to the results of prohibiting these policies. Among the most intriguing issues is whether and how the management of bars can be induced or coerced to issue and support policies restraining the sales incentives of service staff: legal liability and enforcement of control laws by administrative agencies are important possibilities, but the issue requires much more study and experience than are now available.

If the major success story among alcohol-based policies is the national minimum drinking age (MADD, 1991), the fact that large proportions of teenagers continue to consume alcohol and that large (though reduced) proportions of their crash-related fatalities continue to involve impairment suggests the need for effective policies to enforce the law. Research has found that under present circumstances beer is easily purchased in a variety of stores by underage buyers. This situation might be controlled by systematic enforcement of the drinking-age laws through inspections by liquor control agencies. There is considerable room and need for social experimentation and evaluation.

Recommendations based in transportation policy
Among the practical ideas for reducing drunk driving through transportation policy, one policy that is well supported by scientific evidence is discouraging youthful driving, especially during drinking hours. There are likely to be political limits on the implementation of these policies, which require sacrifices of mobility in exchange for safety. A uniform minimum driving age of sixteen, however, corresponding with the practice in the majority of states, would not seem politically unrealistic. In addition, curfews on nighttime driving by youths, perhaps subject to retraction after several months of demonstrated responsible driving (i.e., without reported crashes or violations), seem reasonable. Precedents for this policy exist in several states.

A well-considered proposal for dealing with young people's crash involvement has been offered by Mothers Against Drunk Driving (1991). They propose that the driver's license be granted only to those aged sixteen and older and that for youth between ages sixteen and eighteen there be a curfew on solo driving at night until six months of citation-free driving have been accumulated. No more than one passenger would be permitted in the vehicle driven by a young person during the first twelve months of driving, unless an adult were also present. MADD would also require that, regardless of the general state law, all occupants of cars driven by young people be belted and would suspend licenses until eighteen for a drunk driving offense. This proposal seems a good candidate for adoption and evaluation.

In the absence of considerably more research on existing programs, the negatives and unknowns surrounding policies like safe rides and designated drivers discourage me from strongly endorsing them. I do believe, however, that the time is ripe for a demonstration project subsidizing the use of alternative transportation during drinking hours, with the goal of inducing prospective drivers to arrive at as well as leave drinking establishments by means other than the automobile. In certain cities, a subsidized taxi system might have a reasonable chance of reducing crashes at a feasible cost. The pilot community should be selected with care in order to maximize the attractiveness of the alternative—for instance, a community with an existing fleet of comfortable cabs that are relatively little used at night. The estimated cost of providing the service should be within reason; if a cab ride is to be provided for a modest sum to any address in the city during the target hours, such as after 9 P.M. on weekend nights, a giant metropolis would be impracticable, but a medium-sized city might qualify. I proposed such a program some years ago to a brewer who was looking for opportunities to invest in drunk-driving prevention, but my suggestion was rejected as being unrelated to drunk driving. Perhaps under the dominant paradigm it is. I hope that the suggestion will be better received in the future, as challenging-paradigm thinking takes hold.

Recommendations based in injury control

Injury control offers a wide variety of potential interventions. Many of these promise considerable savings in lives and injuries, but with the disadvantage of having obvious, up-front costs. The highway system, for example, could absorb virtually unlimited amounts of capital investment in straightening curves, installing protective barriers, eliminating conflicting traffic streams, and so forth. In general, the costs associated with such improvements are more than compensated for in increased safety. Likewise, although much has been done to improve the safety of vehicles in recent years, there remain numerous suggestions for vehicle standards that are likely to be cost-effective. Perhaps it suffices to say that although these have been proposed without special reference to the drunk driver, they can reduce alcohol-related deaths as much or very likely more than non-alcohol-related ones. They should not be defined as extraneous to the interests of people concerned with reducing deaths experienced in alcohol-related crashes.

Perhaps the most promising of recent technologies aimed at attenuating the links between impairment and deaths and injuries are passive restraints. These devices are engineered into the vehicle and do not require affirmative action from the occupant in order to be effective. Air bags, for example, are enormously effective in reducing deaths and injuries in frontal crashes. Federal requirements will result in their installation in all new vehicles in the near future. In the short run, however, before the vehicle fleet turns over, they will disproportionately benefit those who need them least. Older vehicles, lacking the new technology, are most likely to be owned by people who drink and drive, who fail to attach their seat belts, and who have crashes. Subsidies, including sales tax rebates, might be considered to encourage drivers to replace older cars with newer, safer ones.

In the absence of universal availability of passive restraints, mandatory seat belt use laws are called for. In the United States, these laws have produced wearing rates of 50 percent. Although lower than the levels achieved in other world jurisdictions, it is considerably higher than rates that prevail in states without such laws. Their enactment should be highly beneficial in preventing injuries and deaths. Since drunk drivers are especially likely to go unbelted, increments in belt wearing are disproportionately beneficial in reducing alcohol-related deaths.

A related recommendation is to enact and enforce mandatory helmet laws for motorcyclists. Violations of helmet use laws are especially easy to observe and prosecute, a fact that has helped such laws achieve among the highest compliance rates known. The relationship between compliance with these laws and reduced cyclist death rates is well demonstrated. The laws can be considered especially relevant to drunk driving inasmuch as FARS data show a high proportion of alcohol-related fatalities among motorcyclists.

The prompt availability of emergency medical services addresses the final link between impaired driving and the loss of life on the highways. Here, as in the case of vehicle and roadway engineering, I merely wish to emphasize that measures aimed at attenuating this link—measures such as the provision of roadside telephones and the funding of helicopter services—should be considered relevant to the drunk driving problem and supported by those who would work to reduce the number of lives lost in alcohol-related crashes. Their utility should, of course, remain subject to disinterested, competent evaluation.

Final remarks

The idea for this book may have originated when I heard Dan Beauchamp (1983) deliver the following message at the crest of dominant paradigm policy making:

"[G]etting even" with drunk drivers doesn't add up to an effective policy for drunk driving. I have no objection to convicted drunk drivers going to jail for their crimes, especially if they are recidivists, or if they have caused the death or the serious injury of another.

Simple justice—not deterrence—supports this shift in policy. But if we really want to prevent drunk driving, we are going to have to cast our nets much wider and take action that is painful to many groups, including the majority of us.

If we are going to save lives currently lost to drunk driving, it will not be enough to redouble our efforts to deter it, even though these efforts be better reasoned and more effective than those of the past. We will have to accept the need to modify social institutions, especially recreation and transportation. As a society we will have to depend somewhat less on the private automobile and indulge somewhat less in our drug of choice, alcohol. If we expect even so that, barring revolutionary changes in our life styles and social institutions, some amount of drunk driving will remain, lives can nonetheless be saved by taking steps that attenuate the links between impairment and error, error and crashes, crashes and injury, and injury and death.

Drunk driving will never be eliminated in a society recognizable as our own. To the individual or family faced with the loss of a loved one, the pain will be as great regardless of the number of fellow sufferers. The citizens' movement has shown how to express this pain in a constructive way, demanding not only justice but also action to prevent others from experiencing it in the future. I hope this review of what is known about drunk driving today will help shift the focus of policy discussion within this movement and elsewhere away from vengeance and toward effective countermeasures. Several kinds of countermeasures exist, countermeasures that include deterrence but go beyond it. Proposals not based on deterrence have sometimes been viewed as irrelevant to drunk driving. In this book I have attempted to demonstrate their relevance.

It is not necessary to discard deterrence of drunk driving as a policy goal. There is scientifically valid evidence that it works. It is not necessary either to discard the demand for justice. No scientific evidence is needed to warrant it. Law and criminal justice can provide useful approaches to confronting the drunk-driving problem. However, if saving lives is to be our primary goal, drunk driving countermeasures based in alcohol policy, transportation policy, and injury reduction as well as deterrence need to be identified, adopted, evaluated, and reformulated in light of the results of the evaluations.

References

Aaron, P., and Musto, D. 1981. Temperance and prohibition in America: A historical overview. In M. Moore and D. Gerstein (eds.), *Alcohol and Public Policy: Beyond the Shadow of Prohibition*. Washington, D.C.: National Academy Press, 127–81.

Ahlstrom, S. 1983. Alcoholics as a problem of alcohol control policy. In P. Golding (ed.), *Alcoholism: Analysis of a World-Wide Problem*. Lancaster, England: MTP Press, 177–89.

Alexander, R., Pons, P., Krischer, J., and Hunt, P. 1984. The effect of advanced life support and sophisticated hospital systems on motor vehicle mortality. *Journal of Trauma* 24: 486–89.

Altshuler, A., Anderson, M., Jones, D., Roos, D., and Womack, J. 1984. *The Future of the Automobile: The Report of MIT's International Automobile Program*. Cambridge: MIT Press.

American Automobile Association. 1990. First a friend, then a host: Party tips and nonalcoholic recipes. Pamphlet.

Andenaes, J. 1974. *Punishment and Deterrence*. Ann Arbor: University of Michigan Press.

Apsler, R. 1989. Transportation alternatives for drinkers. In Office of the Surgeon General, *Surgeon General's Workshop on Drunk Driving: Background Papers*. Rockville, Md.: U.S. Department of Health and Human Services, 157–68.

Apsler, R., Harding, W., and Goldfein, J. 1987. *The Review and Assessment of Designated Driver Programs as an Alcohol Countermeasure Approach*. Technical report. Washington, D.C.: National Highway Traffic Safety Administration.

Armson, R. 1990. *1989 Minnesota State Survey: Results and Technical Report*. Minneapolis: Minnesota Center for Survey Research, University of Minnesota.

Ashley, M. J., and Rankin, J. 1988. A public health approach to the prevention of alcohol-related problems. *Annual Review of Public Health* 9: 233–71.

Association of Erie County Liquor Licensees. N.d. Memorandum in opposition to curtailing hours of operation of legitimate licensed liquor dispensing premises. Unpublished legislative testimony, Buffalo, New York.

Atkin, C. 1989. Mass communication effects on drunk driving. In Office of the Surgeon General, *Surgeon General's Workshop on Drunk Driving: Background Papers*. Rockville, Md.: U.S. Department of Health and Human Services, 1989, 15–34.

Atkin, C., Neuendorf, K., and McDermott, S. 1983. The role of alcohol advertising in excessive and hazardous drinking. *Journal of Drug Education* 13: 313–25.

Babor, T., Mendelson, J., Greenberg, I., and Kuehnle, J. 1978. Experimental analysis of the 'happy hour': Effects of purchase price on alcohol consumption. *Psychopharmacology* 58: 35–41.

Babor, T., Mendelson, J., Uhly, B., and Souza, E. 1980. Drinking patterns in experimental and barroom settings. *Journal of Studies on Alcohol* 41: 635–51.

Barancik, J., Kramer, C., Thode, H., Jr., and Harris, D. 1988. Efficacy of the

New York State seat belt law: Preliminary assessment of occurrence and severity. *Bulletin of the New York Academy of Medicine* 64: 742–49.

Barnes, G., and Welte, J. 1988a. Predictions of driving while intoxicated among teen-agers. *Journal of Drug Issues* 18: 367–84.

———. 1988b. *Alcohol Use and Abuse among Adults in New York State*. Buffalo: New York State Division of Alcoholism and Alcohol Abuse.

Barsby, S., and Associates, Inc. 1988. The economic contribution of the beer industry to the states' economies, 1987. Report prepared for the Beer Institute. Molalla, Oreg.

Baxt, W., and Moody, P. 1983. The impact of a rotorcraft aeromedical emergency car service on trauma mortality. *Journal of the American Medical Association* 249: 3047–51.

Bean, P. 1981. *Punishment*. Oxford: Martin Robertson.

Beauchamp, D. 1983. Beyond MADD: Toward a national policy for drunk driving. Paper presented at the Annual Meeting of the American Association for the Advancement of Science, Detroit.

Beitel, G. A., Sharp, M. C., and Glauz, W. D. 1975. Probability of arrest while driving under the influence of alcohol. *Journal of Studies on Alcohol* 36: 870–76.

Berger, D., and Snortum, J. 1985. Beverage preferences of drinking-driving violators. *Journal of Studies on Alcohol* 46: 232–39.

Berkowitz, A. 1981. *The Effect of Motorcycle Helmet Usage on Head Injuries, and the Effect of Usage Laws on Helmet Wearing Rates*. Technical report. Washington, D.C.: National Highway Traffic Safety Administration.

Best, J. (ed.). 1989. *Images of Issues: Typifying Contemporary Social Problems*. Hawthorne, N.Y.: Aldine.

Birrell, J. 1975. The compulsory breathaliser .05 percent legislation in Victoria. In S. Israelstam and S. Lambert (eds.), *Alcohol, Drugs, and Traffic Safety*. Toronto: Addiction Research Foundation of Ontario, 775–85.

Blomberg, R., Preusser, D., and Ulmer, R. 1987. *Deterrent Effects of Mandatory License Suspension for DWI Convictions*. Technical report. Washington, D.C.: National Highway Traffic Safety Administration.

Blose, J., and Holder, H. 1987a. Public availability of distilled spirits: Structural and reported consumption changes associated with liquor-by-the-drink. *Journal of Studies on Alcohol* 48: 371–79.

———. 1987b. Liquor-by-the-drink and alcohol-related traffic crashes: A natural experiment using time-series analysis. *Journal of Studies on Alcohol* 48: 52–60.

Bota, G., and Cox, J. 1986. Motor vehicle accidents in northeastern Ontario: Are preadmission deaths inevitable? *Canadian Medical Association Journal* 134: 1369–72.

Bragg, B. W., and Cousins, L. S. 1979. Changing the subjective probability of arrest for impaired driving. In I. Johnston (ed.), *Proceedings of the Seventh International Conference on Alcohol, Drugs and Traffic Safety*. Canberra: Australian Government Publishing Service, 649–54.

Brightly, J. M. 1985. The drinking driver: An exploratory study on the deterrent effects of Pennsylvania's driving under the influence legislation. Undergraduate thesis, Pennsylvania State University.

Brodsky, H. 1990. Emergency medical service rescue time in fatal road accidents. *Transportation Research Record* 1270: 89–96.

Buchanan, D., and Lev, J. 1990. *Beer and Fast Cars: How Brewers Target Blue-Collar Youth through Motor Sport Sponsorship*. Washington, D.C.: AAA Foundation for Traffic Safety.

Burns, M., and Moskowitz, H. 1980. *Methods for Estimating Blood Alcohol Concentration*. Technical report. Washington, D.C.: National Highway Traffic Safety Administration.

Campbell, B., and Campbell, F. 1988. Injury reduction and belt use associated with occupant restraint laws. In J. Graham (ed.), *Preventing Automobile Injury: New Findings from Evaluation Research*. Dover, Mass.: Auburn House, 24–50.

Center for Science in the Public Interest. 1989. Legislating under the influence: The booze merchants, money, and Congress. Washington, D.C.: Center for Science in the Public Interest.

———. 1990. Federal beer, wine, and liquor taxes to go up. *Booze News: Updating Advocates on Alcohol Prevention Policies* 2 (5): 1.

Centers for Disease Control. 1990. Alcohol-related mortality and years of life lost—United States, 1987. Morbidity and Mortality Weekly Report, 39 (11): 1–6.

Cleary, J., and Rodgers, A. 1986. *Analysis of the Effects of Recent Changes in Minnesota's DWI Laws*. Part 3: *Longitudinal Analysis of the Policy Impacts*. St. Paul: Research Department, Minnesota House of Representatives.

Cleary, J., Shapiro, E., and Williams, J. 1986. 1985 DWI roadside survey: A preliminary analysis of driver responses to the mail-back questionnaire. St. Paul: Research Department, Minnesota House of Representatives.

Coleman, S., and Guthrie, K. 1988. *Sentencing Effectiveness in Preventing Crime*. St. Paul: Statistical Analysis Center, Minnesota State Planning Agency.

Colman, V., Well, B., and Mosher, J. 1985. Preventing alcohol-related injuries: Dram shop liability in a public health perspective. *Western State Law Review* 12: 417–517.

Collins, J. 1981. *Drinking and Crime*. New York: Guilford Press.

Colon, I. 1983. County-level prohibition and alcohol-related fatal motor vehicle accidents. *Journal of Safety Research* 14: 101–04.

Colon, I., and Cutter, H. 1982. The relationship of beer consumption and state alcohol and motor vehicle policies to fatal accidents. *Journal of Safety Research* 14: 83–89.

Cook, P. 1981. The effect of liquor taxes on drinking, cirrhosis, and auto accidents. In M. Moore and D. Gerstein (eds.), *Alcohol and Public Policy: Beyond the Shadow of Prohibition*. Washington, D.C.: National Academy Press, 255–85.

Cook, P., and Tauchen, G. 1982. The effect of liquor taxes on heavy drinking. *Bell Journal of Economics* 13: 379–90.

Cowan, R., and Mosher, J. (1985). Public health implications of beverage marketing: Alcohol as an ordinary consumer product. *Contemporary Drug Problems* 14: 621–57.

Cowan, T., Robbins, L., and Meszaros, J. 1986. Trial judges' views on driving-under-the-influence laws. *Judges Journal* 24: 4–9, 54–56.

Crandall, R., Gruenspecht, H., Keeler, T., and Lave, L. 1986. *Regulating the Automobile*. Washington, D.C.: Brookings Institution.

Drummond, A. 1986. Driver licensing age and accident involvement rates of young drivers. Road Traffic Authority, Hawthorne, Victoria, Australia.

Dull, R. T., and Giacopassi, D. 1986. An assessment of the effects of alcohol ordinances on selected behaviors and conditions. *Journal of Drug Issues* 16: 511–20.

DuMouchel, W., Williams, A., and Zador, P. 1987. Raising the alcohol purchase age: Its effects on fatal motor vehicle crashes in twenty- six states. *Journal of Legal Studies* 16: 249–66.

Editorial. 1980. Engineering the way through the alcohol haze. *ITE Journal*, November, 12–15.

Enke, K. 1979. Possibilities for improving safety within the driver-vehicle-environment control loop. *Proceedings of the Seventh International Technical Conference on Experimental Safety Vehicles*. Washington, D.C.: Government Printing Office, 789–802.

Epperlein, T. 1985. The use of sobriety checkpoints as a deterrent: An impact assessment. Phoenix: Arizona Department of Public Safety.

Evans, L. 1986. Double pair comparison—a new method to determine how occupant characteristics affect fatality risk in traffic crashes. *Accident Analysis and Prevention* 18: 217–27.

———. 1988. Occupant protection device effectiveness in preventing fatalities. *Proceedings of the Eleventh International Conference on Experimental Safety Vehicles*, 220–27.

———. 1990. The fraction of traffic fatalities attributable to alcohol. *Accident Analysis and Prevention* 22: 587–602.

———. 1991. *Traffic Safety and the Driver*. New York: Van Nostrand Reinhold.

Evans, L., and Frick, M. 1990. *Alcohol's Influence on a Fatality Risk, Given that a Crash Has Occurred*. Technical report. General Motors Research Laboratories.

Evans, L., Frick, M., and Schwing, R. 1990. Is it safer to fly or drive? *Risk Analysis* 10: 239–46.

Falkowski, C. 1984. *The Impact of Two-Day Jail Sentences for Drunk Drivers in Hennepin County, Minnesota*. Final report. Washington, D.C.: National Highway Traffic Safety Administration.

Farrow, J. 1985. Drinking and driving behaviors of 16- to 19-year-olds. *Journal of Studies on Alcohol* 46: 369–74.

———. 1987. Young driver risk taking: A description of dangerous driving situations among 16- to 19-year-old drivers. *International Journal of the Addictions* 22: 1255–67.

Federal Highway Administration. 1988. *Highway Safety Performance—1987: Fatal and Injury Accident Rates on Public Roads in the United States*. Washington, D.C.: U.S. Department of Transportation.

References

———. 1989. *Highway Statistics 1989*. Washington, D.C.: U.S. Department of Transportation.

Fell, J. 1985. *Alcohol Involvement in Fatal Accidents 1980–1984*. Washington, D.C.: National Highway Traffic Safety Administration.

———. 1987. *Alcohol Involvement Rates in Fatal Crashes: A Focus on Young Drivers and Female Drivers*. Washington, D.C.: National Highway Traffic Safety Administration.

Fell, J., and Hertz, E. 1990. Effects of blood alcohol concentration on time of death for fatal crash victims. *Proceedings of the 34th Annual Conference of the Association for the Advancement of Automotive Medicine*, 69–81.

Fell, J., and Nash, C. 1989. The nature of the alcohol problem in U.S. fatal crashes. *Health Education Quarterly* 16: 335–44.

Fingarette, W. 1988. *Heavy Drinking: The Myth of Alcoholism as a Disease*. Berkeley and Los Angeles: University of California Press.

Finkelhor, D., Hotaling, G., and Sedlak, A. 1990. *Missing, Abducted, Runaway, and Thrownaway Children in America: Executive Summary*. Washington, D.C.: U.S. Department of Justice.

"Folklore in Traffic Safety." 1989. *Accident Analysis and Prevention* 21: 103.

Fontaine, R. 1992. DUI pre-arrest alcohol purchases: A survey of Sonoma County drunk-drivers. *Journal of Studies on Alcohol*. In press.

Fortner, G., Oreskovich, M., Copass, M., and Carrico, C. J. 1983. The effects of prehospital trauma care on survival from a 50-meter fall. *Journal of Trauma* 23: 976–81.

Foss, R., Voas, R., Beirness, D., and Wolfe, A. 1990. *Minnesota Road Survey of Drinking and Driving 1990*. St. Paul: Minnesota Department of Public Safety.

Frey, C., Huelke, D., and Gikas, P. 1969. Resuscitation and survival in motor vehicle accidents. *Journal of Trauma* 9: 292–310.

Gans, H. 1979. *Deciding What's News: A Study of CBS Evening News, NBC Nightly News, Newsweek and Time*. New York: Random House.

Geller, E. S., 1983. *Development of Industry-Based Strategies for Motivating Seatbelt Usage*. Blacksburg, Va.: Virginia Polytechnic Institute and State University.

Geller, E. S., and Bigelow, B. 1984. Development of corporate incentive programs for motivating seat belt use: A review. *Traffic Safety Research Review* 3: 21–38.

Geller, E. S., Russ, N., and Altomari, M. 1986. Naturalistic observations of beer drinking among college students. *Journal of Applied Behavior Analysis* 19: 391–96.

General Accounting Office. 1987. *Drinking-Age Laws: An Evaluation Synthesis of Their Impact on Highway Safety*. Report to the Chairman, Subcommittee on Investigations and Oversight, Committee on Public Works and Transportation, House of Representatives. Washington, D.C.: United States General Accounting Office.

General Motors/*Prevention* Magazine Report. 1990. *Auto Safety in America 1990*. Report based on research by Louis Harris & Associates.

Golden, S. 1983. *Driving the Drunk off the Road: A Handbook for Action*. Washington, D.C.: Acropolis Books.

Gordis, E. 1991. From science to social policy: An uncertain road. *Journal of Studies on Alcohol* 52: 101–09.

Grasmick, H., and Bursik, R., Jr. 1990. Conscience, significant others, and rational choice: Extending the deterrence model. *Law and Society Review* 24: 837–61.

Greenfield, L. 1988. *Drunk Driving*. Washington, D.C.: Bureau of Justice Statistics Special Report.

Grossman, Michael. 1988. Health benefits of increases in alcohol and cigarette taxes. Paper presented at the Annual Meeting of the American Economic Association, New York.

Grube, J., and Kearney, K. 1980. *The Yakima County Drinking and Driving Project: An Evaluation of a Mandatory Jail Sentence and a Public Awareness Campaign*. Pullman, Wash.: Social Research Center, Washington State University.

Gusfield, J. 1963. *Symbolic Crusade: Status Politics and the American Temperance Movement*. Urbana: University of Illinois Press.

———. 1981. *The Culture of Public Problems: Drinking-Driving and the Symbolic Order*. Chicago: University of Chicago Press.

———. 1982. Prevention: Rise, decline, and renaissance. In E. Gomberg, H. White, and J. Carpenter (eds.), *Alcohol, Science, and Society Revisited*. Ann Arbor: University of Michigan Press, 402–25.

Gusfield, J., Rasmussen, P., and Kotarba, J. 1984. The social control of drinking-driving: An ethnographic study of bar settings. *Law and Policy* 6: 45–66.

Haddon, W., Jr. 1970. On the escape of tigers: An ecologic note. *American Journal of Public Health* 60: 2229–34.

Haddon, W. 1972. Approaching the reduction of road losses—Replacing guesswork with logic, specificity and scientifically determined fact. Paper presented at the National Road Safety Symposium, Canberra, Australia.

Hagen, R. 1977. *Effectiveness of License Suspension for Drivers Convicted of Multiple DUI Offenses*. Sacramento: California Department of Motor Vehicles.

Hagen, R., Williams, R., McConnell, E., and Fleming, C. 1978. *Suspension and Revocation Effects on the DUI Offender*. Sacramento: California Department of Motor Vehicles.

Hagenzieker, M. 1990. The effects of enforcement and rewards on seat-belt wearing: A field study in the Netherlands. Paper presented at the OECD International Road Safety Symposium, Copenhagen.

Hagge, R., and Marsh, W. 1988. *The Traffic Safety Impact of Provisional Licensing*. Sacramento: Department of Motor Vehicles.

Haight, F. 1983. Road safety: A perspective and a new strategy. Working paper. Pennsylvania State University Transportation Institute. Revised and published under a different title in K. Ogden (ed.), *Traffic Accident Evaluation*. Melbourne, Australia: Monash University.

Hall, J. 1987. Evaluation of wide edgelines. *Transportation Research Record* 1114: 21–27.

Harding, W., Apsler, R., and Goldfein, J. 1988. *The Assessment of Ride Service Programs as an Alcohol Countermeasure*. Technical report. Washington, D.C.: National Highway Traffic Safety Administration.

Hauer, E. 1990. The behaviour of public bodies and the delivery of road safety. Paper presented at the OECD International Road Safety Symposium, Enforcement and Rewarding Strategies and Effects, Copenhagen.

Hauge, R. 1988. The effects of changes in availability of alcoholic beverages. In M. Laurence, J. Snortum, and F. Zimring (eds.), *Social Control of the Drinking Driver*. Chicago: University of Chicago Press, 169–87.

Hause, J. M., Voas, R. B., and Chavez, E. 1980. Conducting voluntary roadside surveys: The Stockton experience. Paper presented at the Satellite Conference to the Eighth International Conference on Alcohol, Drugs, and Traffic Safety, Umeå, Sweden.

Heinzelman, F. 1985. Mandatory confinement as a response to community concerns about drunk driving. *Justice System Journal* 10: 265–78.

Hernandez, A., and Rabow, J. 1987. Passive and assertive student interventions in public and private drunken driving situations. *Journal of Studies on Alcoholism* 48: 269–71.

Highway and Vehicle Safety Report. 1990. National health survey documents increase in safety belt use. (Newsletter) 16 (20): 4.

Highway Safety Foundation. 1972. How much is too much?: A study of problem consumption as related to alcohol and highway safety. Mansfield, Ohio: Highway Safety Foundation.

Hingson, R., Heeren, T., Howland, J., and Winter, M. 1990. Reduced BAC limits for young people (impact on night fatal crashes). Paper presented at the National Conference on Drunk Driving, Washington, D.C.

Hoffman, L. 1973. Alcohol and traffic safety: Screening out the drunken driver. In A. Etzioni and R. Remp (eds.), *Technological Shortcuts to Social Change*. New York: Russell Sage Foundation, 79–101.

Holder, H. 1987. The prevention and reduction of alcohol problems: Public policy and legislation. Paper presented at the National Conference on Alcohol Abuse and Alcoholism, Washington, D.C.

Holder, H., and Blose, J. 1987. Impact of changes in distilled spirits availability on apparent consumption: A time-series analysis of liquor-by-the-drink. *British Journal of Addiction* 82: 623–31.

Homel, R. 1988. *Policing and Punishing the Drinking Driver: A Study of General and Specific Deterrence*. New York: Springer-Verlag.

———. 1990. Random breath testing and random stopping programs in Australia. In R. J. Wilson and R. Mann (eds.), *Drinking and Driving: Advances in Research and Prevention*, New York: Guilford Press, 159–204.

Hooper, F. 1983. The relationship between alcohol control policies and cirrhosis mortality in United States counties. Paper presented at the meeting of the American Public Health Association, Dallas.

Horverak, O. 1989. Availability of sales outlets and optimal prices of alcoholic beverages. Paper presented at the 34th International Institute on the Prevention and Treatment of Alcoholism, Pontault- Combault, France.

Howard-Pitney, B., Johnson, M. D., Altman, D. G., Hopkins, R., and Hammond, N. 1991. Responsible alcohol service: A study of server, manager, and environmental impact. *American Journal of Public Health* 81: 197–98.

IIHS Facts. 1989. *Roadside Hazards*. Arlington, Va.: Insurance Institute for Highway Safety.

Ilich, D. 1986. *The 1982 Driving Under the Influence Laws and the Los Angeles County Municipal Courts: A Three Year Study*. Mimeographed report. Los Angeles: Municipal Courts Planning and Research.

International Taxicab Association. 1990. *Taxicab/Paratransit Fact Book, 1990*. Kensington, Md.: International Taxicab Association.

Irwin, A. 1985. *Risk and the Control of Technology: Public Policies for Road Traffic Safety in Britain and the United States*. Manchester, England: Manchester University Press.

Jacobs, J. 1963. *Death and Life of Great American Cities*. New York: Random House.

Jacobs, J. B. 1989. *Drunk Driving: An American Dilemma*. Chicago: University of Chicago Press.

Jacobs, L., Sinclair, A., Beiser, A., and D'Agostino, R. 1984. Prehospital advanced life support: Benefits in trauma. *Journal of Trauma* 24: 8–13.

Johnson, D. 1986. The effect of administrative license revocation on employment: A preliminary report. Washington, D.C.: National Highway Traffic Safety Administration.

Joksch, H. 1988. *The Impact of Severe Penalties on Drinking and Driving*. Washington, D.C.: AAA Foundation for Traffic Safety.

———. 1991. Does county-level prohibition increase fatal motor vehicle accidents? *Journal of Safety Research* 22: 49–50.

Jolly, D., and Mills, K. 1984. Drinking and driving: The public health problem as a public policy issue. Paper presented at the Annual Meeting of the American Public Health Association, Anaheim, Calif.

Jones, R., Joksch, H., Lacey, J., and Schmidt, H. 1988. *Field Evaluation of Jail Sanctions for DWI*. Technical report. Washington, D.C.: National Highway Traffic Safety Administration.

Jones, R., and Joscelyn, K. 1978. *Alcohol and Highway Safety 1978: A Review of the State of Knowledge*. Washington, D.C.: National Highway Traffic Safety Administration.

Katz, M. 1989. *The Undeserving Poor: From the War on Poverty to the War on Welfare*. New York: Pantheon Books.

Klein, T. 1989. *Changes in Alcohol-Involved Fatal Crashes Associated with Tougher State Alcohol Legislation*. Technical report. Washington, D.C.: National Highway Traffic Safety Administration.

Klitzner, M. 1989. Youth impaired driving: Causes and countermeasures. In Office of the Surgeon General, *Surgeon General's Workshop on Drunk Driving: Back-*

ground Papers. Rockville, Md.: U.S. Department of Health and Human Services, 192–206.

Klitzner, M., Vegega, M., and Gruenewald, P. 1988. An empirical examination of the assumptions underlying youth drinking/driving prevention programs. *Evaluation and Program Planning* 11: 219–35.

Lacey, J., Jones, R., and Stewart, J. 1991. *Cost-Benefit Analysis of Administrative License Suspension*. Technical report. Washington, D.C.: National Highway Traffic Safety Administration.

Lacey, J., Marchetti, L., Stewart, R., Murphy, P., and Jones, R. 1990. *Combining Enforcement and Information to Deter DWI: The Experience of Three Communities*. Chapel Hill: Highway Safety Research Center, University of North Carolina.

Lacey, J., Stewart, R., and Rodgman, E. 1984. *Preliminary Evaluation of the North Carolina Safe Roads Act of 1983*. Chapel Hill: Highway Safety Research Center, University of North Carolina.

Langton, P. 1991. *Drug Use and the Alcohol Dilemma*. Boston: Allyn and Bacon.

Lestina, D., Gloyns, P., and Rattenbury, S. 1990. *Fatally Injured Occupants in Side Impact Crashes*. Arlington, Va.: Insurance Institute for Highway Safety.

Lestina, D., Williams, A., Lund, A., Zador, P., and Kuhlmann, T. 1991. Motor vehicle crash injury patterns and the Virginia seat belt law. *Journal of the American Medical Association* 265: 1409–13.

Levy, D. 1990. Youth and traffic safety: The effects of driving age, experience, and education. *Accident Analysis and Prevention* 22: 327–34.

Lewis, R. 1985. Estimates of DWI recidivism in Minnesota fatal crashes. Unpublished report. St. Paul: Minnesota Criminal Justice System Task Force.

———. 1990. The impact of jail sentences for first time DWI offenders. Unpublished report. St. Paul: Minnesota Criminal Justice System Task Force.

Lowe, M. 1990. Alternatives to the automobile: Transport for liveable cities. Washington, D.C.: Worldwatch Institute.

Lund, A., and Williams, A. 1985. A review of the literature evaluating the Defensive Driving Course. *Accident Analysis and Prevention* 17: 449–60.

Lund, A., and Wolfe, A. 1991. Changes in the incidence of alcohol- impaired driving in the United States, 1973–1986. *Journal of Studies on Alcohol* 52: 293–301.

Lund, A., Zador, P., and Pollner, J. 1987. Motor vehicle occupant fatalities in four states with seat belt use laws. In *Restraint Technologies: Front Seat Occupant Protection*. Warrandale, Penn.: Society of Automotive Engineers, 43–51.

Macdonald, S., and Whitehead, P. 1983. Availability of outlets and consumption of alcoholic beverages. *Journal of Drug Issues* 13: 511–21.

Mackay, M. 1985. Seat belt use under voluntary and mandatory conditions and its effect on casualties. In L. Evans and R. Schwing (eds.), *Human Behavior and Traffic Safety*. New York: Plenum, 259–77.

MADD. 1990. *20 × 2000*. Pamphlet. Irving, Tex.: Mothers Against Drunk Driving.

————. 1991. *Youth Issues Compendium*. Irving, Tex.: Mothers Against Drunk Driving.

Maghsoodloo, S., Brown, D., and Greathouse, P. 1985. Impact of the revision of DUI legislation in Alabama. Manuscript. Department of Industrial Engineering, Auburn University, Alabama.

Mäkelä, K. 1978. Criminalization and punishment in the prevention of alcohol problems. *Contemporary Drug Problems* 5: 327–66.

Mäkelä, K. 1975. Consumption level and cultural drinking patterns as determinants of alcohol problems. *Journal of Drug Issues* 5: 344–57.

————. 1983. The uses of alcohol and their cultural regulation. *Acta Sociologica* 1: 21–31.

Mäkelä, K., Österberg, E., and Sulkunen, P. 1981. Drink in Finland: Increasing alcohol availability in a monopoly state. In E. Single, P. Morgan, and J. de Lint (eds.), *Alcohol, Society and the State. 2: The Social History of Control Policy in Seven Countries*. Toronto: Addiction Research Foundation, 31–60.

Mäkelä, K., Room, R., Single, E., Sulkunen, P., and Walsh, B. 1981. *Alcohol, Society and the State. 1: A Comparative Study of Alcohol Control*. Toronto: Addiction Research Foundation.

Mann, R., and Anglin, L. 1990. Alcohol availability, per capita consumption, and the alcohol-crash problem. In R. J. Wilson and R. Mann (eds.), *Drinking and Driving: Advances in Research and Prevention*. New York: Guilford Press, 205–25.

Manning, W., Keeler, E., Newhouse, J., Sloss, E., and Wasserman, J. 1989. The taxes of sin: Do smokers and drinkers pay their way? *Journal of the American Medical Association* 261: 1604–09.

Martin, S., Annan, S., and Forst, B. 1990. The specific deterrent effects of a jail sanction on first-time drunk drivers: A quasi-experimental study. Unpublished paper. National Institute on Alcohol Abuse and Alcoholism.

Mashaw, J., and Harfst, S. 1990. *The Struggle for Auto Safety*. Cambridge: Harvard University Press.

McCarthy, J. 1990. A media framing context: Its shape, newspaper coverage outcomes and impact upon the citizens' movement against drunken driving. Paper presented at the Workshop on Social Movements, Counterforces and Bystanders, Berlin.

McCarthy, J., Wolfson, M., and Harvey, D. 1987. *Chapter Survey Report of the Project on the Citizens' Movement Against Drunk Driving*. Washington, D.C.: Catholic University, Center for the Study of Youth Development.

McCarthy, J., Wolfson, M., Baker, D., and Mosakowski, E. 1988. The founding of social movement organizations: Local citizens' groups opposing drunken driving. In G. Carroll (ed.), *Ecological Models of Organizations*. Cambridge, Mass.: Ballinger, 71–84.

McCullough, E., Snow, R., Landrum, J., McMillen, D., Anderson, B., Hall, C., Carr, J., and Adams, M. 1990. DUI systems analysis project final report: Component B: Public Awareness. Duplicated report. Mississippi State: Mississippi Alcohol Safety Education Program.

McKnight, A. J. 1988. *Development and Field Test of a Responsible Alcohol Service Program.* Volume 3: *Final Results.* Technical report. Washington, D.C.: National Highway Traffic Safety Administration.

McKnight, A. J., Hyle, P., and Albrecht, L. 1983. *Youth License Control Demonstration Project.* Technical report. Washington, D.C.: National Highway Traffic Safety Administration.

McKnight, A. J., and Marques, P. 1990. *Host and Server Determination of Alcohol Intoxication Level.* Technical report. Washington, D.C.: National Highway Traffic Safety Administration.

McKnight, A. J., and Voas, R. 1990. The effect of license suspension upon DWI recidivism. *Alcohol, Drugs and Driving* 6: 1–12.

Meier, S., Brigham, T., and Handel, G. 1984. Effects of feedback on legally intoxicated drivers. *Journal of Studies on Alcohol* 45: 528–33.

Mercer, W. 1985. The relationship among driving while impaired charges, police drinking-driving roadcheck activity, media coverage, and alcohol-related casualty traffic accidents. *Accident Analysis and Prevention* 17: 467–74.

Misner, R., and Ward, P. 1975. Severe penalties for driving offenses: Deterrence analysis. *Arizona State Law Journal* 1975: 677–713.

Montague, W. 1989. Drunk driving foes accept big gifts from alcoholic-beverage producers. *Chronicle of Philanthropy* 1: 1, 12–14.

Moore, M., and Gerstein, D. (eds.). 1981. *Alcohol and Public Policy: Beyond the Shadow of Prohibition.* Washington, D.C.: National Academy Press.

Morrall, J., III. 1986. A review of the record. *Regulation* 10: 25–34.

Morse, B., and Elliott, D. 1990. Hamilton County drinking and driving study: 30-month report. Manuscript. Institute of Behavioral Science, University of Colorado, Boulder.

Mosher, J., and Wallack, L. 1989. Proposed reforms in the regulation of alcoholic beverage advertising. *Contemporary Drug Problems* 8: 87–106.

Moskowitz, H., and Burns, M. 1990. Effects of alcohol on driving performance. *Alcohol Health and Research World* 14: 12–14.

Moskowitz, H., and Robinson, C. 1988. Effects of low doses of alcohol on driving-related skills: A review of the evidence. Technical report. Washington, D.C.: National Highway Traffic Safety Administration.

Motor Vehicles Manufacturers Association. 1989. *MVMA Motor Vehicle Facts & Figures '89.* Detroit: Motor Vehicles Manufacturers Association.

National Alcohol Tax Coalition. 1989. *Impact of Alcohol Excise Tax Increases on Federal Revenues, Alcohol Consumption and Alcohol Problems.* Washington, D.C.: Center for Science in the Public Interest.

National Center for Statistics and Analysis. 1990a. Drunk driving facts. Bulletin. Washington, D.C.: National Highway Traffic Safety Administration.

———. 1990b. *Occupant Protection Facts.* Washington, D.C.: National Highway Traffic Safety Administration.

National Commission on Drug-Free Schools. 1990. *Toward a Drug-Free Generation: A Nation's Responsibility.* Final report..Washington, D.C.: National Commission on Drug-Free Schools.

National Highway Traffic Safety Administration. 1983. *The Use of Safety Checkpoints for DWI Enforcement.* Washington, D.C.: National Highway Traffic Safety Administration.

———. 1984. Federal motor vehicle safety standard: Occupant crash protection. *Federal Register* 49: 28962–29010.

———. 1989. *Fatal Accident Reporting System 1988.* Washington, D.C.: U.S. Department of Transportation.

———. 1990. *Highway Safety Priority Plan: Moving America into the 21st Century.* Washington, D.C.: U.S. Department of Transportation.

———. 1991. *Potential Lives Saved If Administrative License Revocation Adopted.* Mimeograph. Washington, D.C.: National Highway Traffic Safety Administration.

National Institute on Alcohol Abuse and Alcoholism. 1989. *The Epidemiology of Alcohol Use and Abuse among U.S. Minorities.* Washington, D.C.: Government Printing Office.

———. 1990. *Alcohol and Health.* Rockville, Md.: U.S. Department of Health and Human Services.

Nedas, N., Balcar, G., and Macy, P. 1982. Road markings as an alcohol countermeasure for highway safety: Field study of standard and wide edgelines. *Transportation Research Record* 847: 43–46.

Neuman, C., and Rabow, J. 1986. Drinkers' use of physical availability of alcohol: Buying habits and consumption level. *International Journal of the Addictions* 20: 1663–73.

New York Times. December 15, 1988. Page A 34.

Nichols, J. 1990. Treatment versus deterrence. *Alcohol Health and Research World* 14: 44–51.

Nichols, J., Ellingstad, V., and Reis, R. 1980. The effectiveness of education and treatment programs for drinking drivers: A decade of evaluation. Paper presented at the International Conference on Alcohol, Drugs, and Traffic Safety, Stockholm, Sweden.

Nichols, J., and Ross, H. L. 1989. The effectiveness of legal sanctions in dealing with drinking drivers. In Office of the Surgeon General, *Surgeon General's Workshop on Drunk Driving: Background Papers.* Rockville, Md.: U.S. Department of Health and Human Services, 93–112.

———. 1990. The effectiveness of legal sanctions in dealing with drinking drivers. *Alcohol, Drugs, and Driving* 6: 33–60.

Nichols, J., and Shinar, D. 1990. Driver characteristics and impairment: Implications for behavioral and environmental countermeasures. Mimeographed paper. Washington, D.C.: National Highway Traffic Safety Administration.

O'Connor, P. 1986. Report on graduated driver licensing and other road accident countermeasures focusing on young drivers. Mimeographed report. Road Safety Division, Adelaide, South Australia.

O'Day, J., and Filkins, L. 1983. Attitudes toward wearing belts: A survey of Michigan drivers. *UMTRI Research Review* 14: 1–12.

O'Donnell, M. 1985. Research on drinking locations of alcohol-impaired drivers: Implications for prevention policies. *Journal of Public Health Policy* 6: 510–25.

Office of the Surgeon General. 1989. *Surgeon General's Workshop on Drunk Driving: Proceedings*. Rockville, Md.: U.S. Department of Health and Human Services.

Ornstein, S., and Levy, D. 1983. Price and income elasticities of demand for alcoholic beverages. In M. Galanter (ed.), *Recent Developments in Alcoholism*. New York: Plenum, 303–45.

Ostrom, M., Huelke, D., Waller, P., Eriksson, A., and Blow, F. 1991. Some biases in the alcohol investigative process in traffic fatalities. Manuscript. Ann Arbor: University of Michigan Transportation Research Institute.

Packer, H. 1968. *The Limits of the Criminal Sanction*. Stanford: Stanford University Press.

Palmer, J., and Tix, P. 1985. Minnesota alcohol roadside survey. St. Cloud, Minn.: St. Cloud State University.

Partyka, M. 1988a. Belt effectiveness in fatal accidents. In M. Partyka, *Papers on adult seat belts: Effectiveness and use*. Technical report. Washington, D.C.: National Highway Traffic Safety Administration, 79–84.

———. 1988b. Lives saved by child restraints from 1982 through 1987. Technical report. Washington, D.C.: National Highway Traffic Safety Administration.

Perchonok, K., Ranney, T., Baum, A. S., Morris, D., and Eppich, J. 1978. *Hazardous Effects of Highway Features and Roadside Objects*. Technical report. Washington, D.C.: Federal Highway Administration.

Perper, J., Twerski, A., and Wienand, J. 1986. Tolerance at high blood alcohol concentrations: A study of 220 cases and review of the literature. *Journal of Forensic Sciences* 31: 212–21.

Perrine, M. W., and Foss, R. 1990. *The 1990 Roadside Survey of Drinking and Driving in Northeastern Ohio*. North Canton, Ohio: Human Ecology Institute.

Phelps, C. 1988. Alcohol taxes and highway safety. In J. Graham (ed.), *Preventing Automobile Injury: New Findings from Evaluation Research*. Dover, Mass.: Auburn House, 197–219.

Popkin, C., Li, L., Lacey, J., Stewart, R., and Waller, P. 1983. *An Initial Evaluation of the North Carolina Alcohol and Drug Education Traffic Schools*. Volume 1. Chapel Hill: Highway Safety Research Center, University of North Carolina.

Popkin, C., Stewart, J., and Lacey, J. 1988. *A Follow-Up Evaluation of North Carolina's Alcohol and Drug Education Traffic Schools and Mandatory Substance Abuse Assessments: Final Report*. Chapel Hill: Highway Safety Research Center, University of North Carolina.

Postman, N., Nystrom, C., State, L., and Weingartner, C. 1987. *Myths, Men and*

Beer: An Analysis of Beer Commercials on Broadcast TV. Washington, D.C.: AAA Foundation for Traffic Safety.

Presidential Commission on Drunk Driving. 1983. *Final Report*. Washington, D.C.: Presidential Commission on Drunk Driving.

Preusser, D., and Williams, A. 1991. Sales of alcohol to underage purchasers in three New York counties and Washington, D.C. Arlington, Va.: Insurance Institute for Highway Safety.

Preusser, D., Williams, A., and Lund, A. 1986. Seat belt use among New York bar patrons. *Journal of Public Health Policy* 7: 470–79.

Preusser, D., Williams, A., and Zador, P. 1984. The effect of curfew laws on motor vehicle crashes. *Law and Policy* 6: 115–28.

Rabow, J., and Watts, R. 1982. Alcohol availability, alcoholic beverage sales and alcohol-related problems. *Journal of Studies on Alcohol* 43: 767–801.

Reinarman, C. 1988. The social construction of an alcohol problem: The case of Mothers Against Drunk Drivers and social control in the 1980s. *Theory and Society* 17: 91–120.

Reinfurt, D., Campbell, B., Stewart, J. R., and Stutts, J. 1988. *North Carolina's Occupant Restraint Law: A Three Year Evaluation*. Chapel Hill: Highway Safety Research Center, University of North Carolina.

Retting, R., 1991. *Improving Urban Traffic Safety: A Multidisciplinary Approach*. Privately printed brochure, funded by the Volvo Car Corporation.

Robbins, L. 1986. Driving-under-the-influence of alcohol and drugs: The judge's role. Paper presented at the National Conference on DWI Recidivism of the National Commission Against Drunk Driving. Atlanta.

Robertson, L., 1980. Engineering for people versus people engineering. Paper presented at the Annual Meeting of the American Public Health Association, Detroit.

———. 1981. Automobile safety regulations and death reductions in the United States. *American Journal of Public Health* 71: 818–22.

Robertson, L., Kelley, A., O'Neill, B., Wixom, C., Eiswirth, R., and Haddon, W., Jr. 1974. A controlled study of the effect of television messages on safety belt use. *American Journal of Public Health* 64: 1071–81.

Robertson, L., Rich, R., and Ross, H. L. 1973. Jail sentences for driving while intoxicated in Chicago: A judicial policy that failed. *Law and Society Review* 8: 55–67.

Rodgers, A. 1990. Preliminary report on DWI recidivism from the Vanhon database: Trends from the update of the 1983 study. St. Paul: Minnesota Department of Public Safety.

Room, R. 1978. Evaluating the effect of drinking laws on drinking. In J. Ewing and B. Rouse (eds.), *Drinking: Alcohol in American Society—Issues and Current Research*. Chicago: Nelson-Hall, 267–89.

———. 1984. Alcohol control and public health. *Annual Review of Public Health* 5: 293–317.

Ross, H. L. 1975. The Scandinavian myth: The effectiveness of drinking and driving legislation in Sweden and Norway. *Journal of Legal Studies* 4: 1–78.

———. 1976. The neutralization of severe penalties: Some traffic law studies. *Law and Society Review* 10: 403–13.

———. 1977. Deterrence regained: The Cheshire Constabulary's "breathaliser blitz." *Journal of Legal Studies* 6: 241–49.

———. 1982. *Deterring the Drinking Driver: Legal Policy and Social Control.* Lexington, Mass.: D. C. Heath Lexington Books.

———. 1986. The brewing industry views the drunk-driving problem. *Accident Analysis and Prevention* 18: 495–504.

———. 1987a. Administrative license revocation in New Mexico: An evaluation. *Law and Policy* 9: 6–16.

———. 1987b. Reflections on doing policy-relevant sociology: How to cope with MADD mothers. *The American Sociologist* 18: 173–78.

———. 1991. *Administrative License Revocation for Drunk Drivers: Options and Choices in Three States.* Washington, D.C.: AAA Foundation for Traffic Safety.

Ross, H. L., and Foley, J. 1987. Judicial disobedience of the mandate to imprison drunk drivers. *Law and Society Review* 21: 315–23.

Ross, H. L., and Gonzales, P. 1988. The effect of license revocation on drunk-driving offenders. *Accident Analysis and Prevention* 20: 379–91.

Ross, H. L., Howard, J., Ganikos, M., and Taylor, E. 1991. Drunk driving among American blacks and Hispanics. *Accident Analysis and Prevention* 23: 1–11.

Ross, H. L., and LaFree, G. 1986. Deterrence in criminology and social policy. In N. Smelser and D. Gerstein (eds.), *Behavioral and Social Science: Fifty Years of Discovery.* Washington, D.C.: National Academy Press, 129–51.

Ross, H. L., McCleary, R., and LaFree, G. 1990. Can the threat of jail deter drunk drivers? The Arizona case. *Journal of Criminal Law and Criminology* 81: 156–70.

Ross, H. L., and Voas, R. B. 1989. *The New Philadelphia Story: The Effects of Severe Punishment for Drunk Driving.* Washington, D.C.: AAA Foundation for Traffic Safety.

Rush, B., Gliksman, L., and Brook, R. 1986. Alcohol availability, alcohol consumption, and alcohol-related damage: The distribution of consumption model. *Journal of Studies on Alcohol* 47: 1–10.

Russ, N., and Geller, E. S. 1987. Training bar personnel to prevent drunken driving: A field evaluation. *American Journal of Public Health* 77: 952–54.

Sadler, D., and Perrine, M. 1984. *An Evaluation of the California Drunk Driving Countermeasure System.* Volume 2: *The Long-Term Traffic Safety Impact of a Pilot Alcohol Abuse Treatment as an Alternative to License Suspensions.* Sacramento: California Department of Motor Vehicles.

Saffer, H., and Grossman, M. 1987a. Drinking age laws and highway mortality rates: Cause and effect. *Economic Inquiry* 25: 403–17.

———. 1987b. Beer taxes, the legal drinking age, and youth motor vehicle fatalities. *Journal of Legal Studies* 16: 351–74.

Saltz, R. 1989. Server intervention and responsible beverage service programs. In Office of the Surgeon General, *Surgeon General's Workshop on Drunk Driving: Background Papers*. Rockville, Md.: U.S. Department of Health and Human Services, 169–79.

Salzberg, R., and Klingberg, C. 1983. The effectiveness of deferred prosecution for driving while intoxicated. *Journal of Studies on Alcohol* 44: 299–306.

Schmidt, A. 1989. Electronic monitoring of offenders increases. *NIJ Reports* No. 212.

Schneider, K. 1971. *Autokind vs. Mankind: An Analysis of Tyranny, a Proposal for Rebellion, a Plan for Reconstruction*. New York: W. W. Norton.

Schudson, M. 1984. *Advertising, the Uneasy Persuasion: Its Dubious Impact on American Society*. New York: Basic Books.

Schwing, R. 1987. Finding the benefits of safer vehicles. Paper presented at the Annual Meeting of the American Association for the Advancement of Science.

Segars, L., and Ryan, M. 1986. Survey of off-site purchase and consumption locations of convicted drinking drivers. Unpublished report. San Diego County Department of Health Services.

Shinar, D., and Fell, J. 1990. The effects of raised lane markers on the accident involvement of older and alcohol-impaired drivers. Paper presented at the Annual Meeting of the Human Factors Society, Orlando, Fla.

Siegal, H. 1985. *Impact of Driver Intervention Program on DWI Recidivism and Problem Drinking*. Washington, D.C.: National Highway Traffic Safety Administration.

Single, E. 1991. The availability theory of alcohol-related problems. In C. Chaudron and D. Wilkinson (eds.), *Theories on Alcoholism*. Toronto: Addiction Research Foundation of Ontario, 325–52.

Sivak, M., Weintraub, D., and Flannagan, M. 1991. Nonstop flying is safer than driving. *Risk Analysis* 11: 145–48.

Skinner, D., and Hoxie, P. 1988. *Effects of Seatbelt Laws on Highway Fatalities: Update—April 1988*. Technical report. Washington, D.C.: National Highway Traffic Safety Administration.

Slovenko, R. 1983. The torture of the automobile way of life, *Medicine and Law* 2: 385–98.

Slovic, R., Fischhoff, B., and Lichtenstein, S. 1978. Accident probabilities and seat belt usage: A psychological perspective. *Accident Analysis and Prevention* 10: 281–85.

Smart, R. 1977. The relationship of availability of alcoholic beverages to per capita consumption and alcoholism rates. *Journal of Studies on Alcohol* 38: 891–96.

———. 1988. Does alcohol advertising affect overall consumption? A review of empirical studies. *Journal of Studies on Alcohol* 49: 314–23.

Smart, R., and Adlaf, E. 1986. Banning happy hours: The impact on drinking and impaired driving charges in Ontario, Canada. *Journal of Studies on Alcohol* 47: 256–58.

Snortum, J. 1988. Deterrence of alcohol-impaired driving: An effect in search of a cause. In M. Laurence, J. Snortum, and F. Zimring (eds.), *Social Control of the Drinking Driver*. Chicago: University of Chicago Press, 189–226.

Snortum, J., Kremer, L., and Berger, D. 1987. Alcoholic beverage preference as a public statement: Self-concept and social image of college drinkers. *Journal of Studies on Alcohol* 48: 243–51.

Snortum, J., Hauge, R., and Berger, D. 1986. Deterring alcohol-impaired driving: A comparative analysis of compliance in Norway and the United States. *Justice Quarterly* 3: 139–65.

Spector, M., and Kitsuse, J. 1987. *Constructing Social Problems*. Hawthorne, N.Y.: Aldine De Gruyter.

Speiglman, R., and Goetz, B. 1987. The public health implications of alcohol availability: An analytic critique. Unpublished paper. Berkeley, Calif.: Alcohol Research Group.

States, J., Annechiarico, R., Good, R., Lieou, J., Andrews, M., Cushman, L., and Ingersoll, G. 1990. A time comparison study of the New York State safety belt use law utilizing hospital admission and police accident report information. *Accident Analysis and Prevention* 22: 509–22.

Steinbock, N. 1985. Drunk driving. *Philosophy and Public Affairs* 14: 278–95.

Stewart, K., and Ellingstad, V. 1989. Rehabilitation countermeasures for drinking drivers. In Office of the Surgeon General, *Surgeon General's Workshop on Drunk Driving: Background Papers*. Rockville, Md.: U.S. Department of Health and Human Services, 234–46.

Stewart, K., Gruenewald, P., and Roth, T. 1989. *An Evaluation of Administrative Per Se Laws*. Final report. Washington, D.C.: National Institute of Justice.

Stitt, B. G., and Giacopassi, D. 1990. Alcohol availability and alcohol-related crime. Unpublished paper. University of Nevada, Reno.

Strand, G., and Garr, M. 1990. Driving under the influence and low self-control: A test of a general theory of crime. Paper presented at the Annual Meeting of the American Society of Criminology, Baltimore.

Stutts, J., Hunter, W., and Campbell, B. 1984. Three studies evaluating the effectiveness of incentives for increasing safety belt use. *Traffic Safety Evaluation Reasearch Review* 3: 9–20.

Summers, L., and Harris, D. 1978. *The General Deterrence of Driving While Intoxicated*. Technical report. Washington, D.C.: National Highway Traffic Safety Administration.

Tashima, H., and Marelich, W. 1989. *A Comparison of the Relative Effectiveness of Alternative Sanctions for DUI Offenders*. Sacramento: California Department of Motor Vehicles.

Tashima, H., and Peck, R. 1986. *An Evaluation of the California Drunk Driving Countermeasure System*. Volume 3: *An Evaluation of the Specific Deterrent Effects of Alternative Sanctions for First and Repeat Offenders*. Sacramento: California Department of Motor Vehicles.

Terhune, K., and Fell, J. 1982. *The Role of Alcohol, Marijuana and Other Drugs in the Accidents of Injured Drivers*. Technical report. Washington, D.C.: National Highway Traffic Safety Administration.

Tittle, C., and Rowe, A. 1974. Certainty of arrest and crime rates: A further test of the deterrence hypothesis. *Social Forces* 52: 455–61.

Toxic Substances Board. 1989a. *Health or Tobacco: An End to Tobacco Advertising and Promotion*. Wellington, New Zealand: Government Printing Office.

———. 1989b. *A Reply to Tobacco Industry Claims about Health or Tobacco*. Wellington, New Zealand: Government Printing Office.

Transportation Research Board, National Research Council. 1984. *55: A Decade of Experience*. Washington, D.C.: National Academy of Science.

———. 1987. *Zero Alcohol and Other Options: Limits for Truck and Bus Drivers*. Washington, D.C.: National Research Council.

Treat, J. 1980. A study of precrash factors involved in traffic accidents. *HSRI Research Review* 10–11: 1–35.

Trinca, G., Johnston, I., Campbell, B., Haight, F., Knight, P., Mackay, M., McLean, J., and Petrucelli, E. 1988. *Reducing Traffic Injury: A Global Challenge*. Melbourne: Royal Australasian College of Surgeons.

Ungerleider, S., and Bloch, S. 1988. Perceived effectiveness of drinking-driving countermeasures: An evaluation of MADD. *Journal of Studies on Alcohol* 49: 191–95.

U.S. Congress. 1968. *Alcohol and Highway Safety*. Washington, D.C.: Government Printing Office.

U.S. Department of Commerce. 1989. *1989 U.S. Industrial Outlook*. Washington, D.C.: Government Printing Office.

U.S. Department of Health and Human Services. 1990. *Alcohol and Health: Seventh Special Report to the U.S. Congress from the Secretary of Health and Human Services*. Rockville, Md.: National Institute on Alcohol Abuse and Alcoholism.

U.S. Department of Transportation. 1980. *A Report to the Congress on the Effect of Motorcycle Helmet Use Law Repeal—A Case for Helmet Use*. Washington, D.C.: National Highway Traffic Safety Administration.

U.S. General Accounting Office. 1976. *Effectiveness, Benefits, and Costs of Federal Safety Standards for Protection of Passenger Car Occupants*. Report to the Committee on Commerce, United States Senate, by the Comptroller General of the United States. Washington, D.C.: General Accounting Office.

Van Houten, R., Nau, P., and Jonah, B. 1983. Effects of feedback on impaired driving. In S. Kaye and G. Meier (eds.), *Alcohol, Drugs and Traffic Safety: Proceedings of the Ninth International Conference on Alcohol, Drugs and Traffic Safety—San Juan, Puerto Rico, 1983*. Washington, D.C.: U.S. Department of Transportation, 1375–94.

Vargus, B. 1985. If I do I might get caught, but I doubt it. Unpublished report. Public Opinion Laboratory, Indiana University-Purdue University, Indianapolis.

Vingilis, E., Mann, R., Gavin, D., Adlaf, E., and Anglin, L. 1990. Effects of sentence severity on drinking driving offenders. *Alcohol, Drugs and Driving* 6: 189–97.

Voas, R. 1975. A systems approach to the development and evaluation of countermeasures programs for the drinking driver. In M. Chafetz (ed.), *Proceedings of the Fourth Annual Alcoholism Conference of the National Institute of Alcohol Abuse and Alcoholism*. Washington, D.C.: U.S. Department of Health, Education, and Welfare, 28–49.

———. 1986. Evaluation of jail as a penalty for drunk driving. *Alcohol, Drugs, and Driving* 2: 47–70.

———. 1988a. Comments. In J. Graham (ed.), *Preventing Automobile Injury: New Findings from Evaluation Research*. Dover, Mass.: Auburn House, 188–96.

———. 1988b. Emerging technologies for controlling the drunk driver. In M. Laurence, J. Snortum, and F. Zimring (eds.), *Social Control of the Drinking Driver*. Chicago: University of Chicago Press, 321–70.

———. 1991. Actions against vehicles and vehicle tags to reduce driving while suspended. Executive summary, mimeographed report. Landover, Md.: National Public Services Research Institute.

Voas, R. B., and Hause, J. 1983. *Deterring the Drinking Driver: The Stockton Experience*. Alexandria, Va.: National Public Services Research Institute.

Voas, R. B., and Lacey, J. 1989. Issues in the enforcement of impaired driving laws in the United States. In Office of the Surgeon General, *Surgeon General's Workshop on Drunk Driving: Working Papers*. Rockville, Md.: U.S. Department of Health and Human Services, 136–56.

Voas, R. B., Rhodenizer, E., and Lynn, C. 1985. *Evaluation of Charlottesville Checkpoint Operations*. Technical report. Washington, D.C.: National Highway Traffic Safety Administration.

Wagenaar, A. 1981. Effects of the raised legal drinking age on motor vehicle accidents in Michigan. *HSRI Research Review* 11 (4): 1–8.

———. 1983. *Alcohol, Young Drivers, and Traffic Accidents*. Lexington, Mass.: D. C. Heath Lexington Books.

Wagenaar, A., and Farrell, S. 1989. Alcohol beverage control policies: Their role in preventing alcohol-impaired driving. In Office of the Surgeon General, *Surgeon General's Workshop on Drunk Driving: Background Papers*. Rockville, Md.: U.S. Department of Health and Human Services, 1–14.

Wagenaar, A., and Holder, H. 1990. Changing from public to private sale of wine: Results from natural experiments in the United States. Unpublished paper. Berkeley, Calif.: Prevention Research Center.

Wagenaar, A., Molnar, L., Streff, S., and Schultz, R. 1988. *Michigan Omnibus State Safety Survey: Fall, 1987*. Ann Arbor: University of Michigan Transportation Research Institute.

Wagenaar, A., and O'Malley, P. 1990. The legal drinking age of 21 in the United States: Effects on drinking practices, risky behaviors, and traffic clashes. Paper presented at the 18th International Institution on the Prevention and Treatment of Drug Dependence, Berlin.

Wagenaar, A., Streff, F., and Maybee, R. 1987. *Michigan Omnibus State Safety Survey: Summer, 1987.* Ann Arbor: University of Michigan Transportation Research Institute.

Wagenaar, A., Streff, F., and Schultz, R. 1990. Effects of the 65 mph speed limit on injury morbidity and mortality. *Accident Analysis and Prevention* 22: 571–86.

Wagenaar, A., and Webster, D. 1985. Effects of Michigan's mandatory child restraint law. *UMTI Research Review* 15: 1–15.

Wagenaar, A., and Wiviott, M. 1985. *Direct Observation of Seat Belt Use in Michigan: July 1985.* Ann Arbor: University of Michigan Transportation Research Institute.

Wall Street Journal. 1983. Many have driven while drunk. Section 2, p. 27 (Western Edition), October 31, 1983.

Wallack, L., Cassady, D., and Grube, J. 1990. *TV Beer Commercials and Children: Exposure, Attention, Beliefs, and Expectations about Drinking as an Adult.* Washington, D.C.: AAA Foundation for Traffic Safety.

Walsh, D. 1991. Electronics and vehicle safety. *Automotive Engineering* 99 (3), 23–25.

Ward, A. 1987. Discussion. *Transportation Research Record* 1114: 28–29.

Warner, K. 1989. Effects of the antismoking campaign: An update. *American Journal of Public Health* 79: 144–51.

Watson, G., Zador, P., and Wilks, A. 1981. Helmet use, helmet use laws, and motorcyclist fatalities. *American Journal of Public Health* 71: 297–300.

Wechsler, H., and Isaac, N. 1991. *Alcohol and the College Freshman: "Binge" Drinking and Associated Problems.* Washington, D.C.: AAA Foundation for Traffic Safety.

Weed, F. 1985. Grass-roots activism and the drunk-driving issue: A survey of MADD chapters. Paper presented at the Annual Meeting of the American Sociological Association, Washington, D.C.

Wells, J., Williams, A., and Fields, M. 1989. Coverage gaps in seat belt use laws. *American Journal of Public Health* 79: 332–33.

Wells-Parker, E., and Cosby, P. 1987. *Impact of a Driver's License Suspension on Employment Stability of Drunken Drivers.* Mississippi State: Mississippi State University Social Science Research Center.

West, J., Trunkey, D., and Lim, R. 1979. Systems of trauma care: A study of two counties. *Archives of Surgery* 114: 455–60.

Wieczorek, W., Miller, B., and Nochajski, T. 1989. Bar versus home drinkers: Different subgroups of problem-drinker drivers. Research Note 89–6, New York State Division of Alcoholism and Alcohol Abuse.

Williams, A. 1985. Fatal motor vehicle crashes involving teenagers. *Pediatrician* 12: 37–40.

———. 1987. Effective and ineffective policies for reducing injuries associated with youthful drivers. *Alcohol, Drugs, and Driving* 3: 109–17.

———. 1989. *Alcohol-Impaired Driving: The Problem and Some Countermeasures.* Arlington, Va.: Insurance Institute for Highway Safety.

———. 1991. The 1980s decline in alcohol impaired driving and crashes and why it occurred. Paper presented at the International Symposium on Problems with DWI Arrests, Convictions, and Sentencing, Santa Monica, Calif.

Williams, A., Karpf, R., and Zador, P. 1984. Variations in minimum licensing age and fatal motor vehicle crashes. *American Journal of Public Health* 73: 1401–04.

Williams, A., and Lund, A. 1984. Deterrent effects of roadblocks on drinking and driving. *Traffic Safety Evaluation Research Review* 3: 7–18.

———. 1986. Adults' views of laws that limit teenagers' driving and access to alcohol. *Journal of Public Health Policy* 7: 190–97.

———. 1988. Mandatory seat-belt use laws and occupant crash protection in the United States: Present status and future prospects. In J. Graham (ed.), *Preventing Automobile Injury: New Findings from Evaluation Research*. Dover, Mass.: Auburn House, 51–72.

Williams, A., Wells, J., Lund, A., and Teed, N. 1990. Seat belt use in cars with automatic belts. *American Journal of Public Health* 80: 1514–16.

Williams, A., Zador, P., Harris, S., and Karpf, R. 1983. The effect of raising the legal minimum drinking age on involvement in fatal crashes. *Journal of Legal Studies* 12: 169–79.

Williams, G., DuFour, M., and Bertolucci, D. 1986. Drinking levels, knowledge, and associated characteristics, 1985 NHIS findings. *Public Health Reports* 181: 593–98.

Wilson, D. 1989. *The Effectiveness of Motorcycle Helmets in Preventing Fatalities*. Technical report. Washington, D.C.: National Highway Traffic Safety Administration.

Wiseman, J. 1979. *Stations of the Lost: The Treatment of Skid Row Alcoholics*. Chicago: University of Chicago Press.

Wittman, F. 1986. Local control of alcohol availability to prevent alcohol problems: Challenges for city and county planners. Mimeographed paper. Berkeley, Calif.: Prevention Research Center.

Wolfe, A. 1973. 1973 U.S. national roadside breathtesting survey: Procedures and results. Ann Arbor: University of Michigan Highway Safety Research Institute.

Wright, P., Hall, J., and Zador, P. 1983. Low-cost countermeasures for ameliorating run-off-the-road crashes. *Transportation Research Record* 926: 1–7.

Zador, P. 1991. Alcohol-related risk of fatal driver injuries in relation to driver age and sex. *Journal of Studies on Alcohol* 52: 302–10.

Zador, P., Lund, A., Fields, M., and Weinberg, K. 1989. Fatal crash involvement and laws against alcohol-impaired driving. *Journal of Public Health Policy* 10: 467–85.

Zador, P., Stein, H., Wright, P., and Hall, J. 1987. Effects of chevrons, postmounted delineators, and raised pavement markers on driver behavior at roadway curves. *Transportation Research Record* 1114: 1–10.

Zador, P., Wright, P., and Karpf, R. 1982. Effect of pavement markers on nighttime crashes in Georgia. Arlington, Va.: Insurance Institute for Highway Safety.

Zimring, F., and Hawkins, G. 1973. *Deterrence: The Legal Threat in Crime Control.* Chicago: University of Chicago Press.

Zylman, R. 1974. A critical evaluation of the literature on alcohol involvement in highway deaths. *Accident Analysis and Prevention* 6: 163–204.

Index